Gaining
PERSPECTIVE
Through Cancer

DAVID GAST

Sequel to *Musing and Muttering Through Cancer*

Gaining Perspective Through Cancer
Copyright © 2013 by David Gast

Scripture taken from the HOLY BIBLE, NEW INTERNATIONAL VERSION ®. Copyright ©1973, 1978, 1984, 2011 by Biblica Inc™. Used by permission of Zondervan Publishing House. All rights reserved worldwide. The "NIV" and "New International Version" trademarks are registered in the United States Patent and Trademark Office by Biblica Inc™. Use of either trademark requires the permission of International Bible Society. Scripture quotations marked "NLT" are taken from the Holy Bible, New Living Translation. Copyright 1996. Used by permission of Tyndale House Publishing, Inc., Wheaton, Illinois 60189. All rights reserved.

ISBN: 978-1-77069-974-8

Printed in Canada

Word Alive Press
131 Cordite Road, Winnipeg, MB R3W 1S1
www.wordalivepress.ca

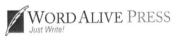

WORD ALIVE PRESS
Just Write!

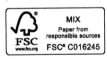

MIX
Paper from
responsible sources
FSC
www.fsc.org   FSC® C016245

Dedication

I dedicate this book to you, Sharon, my loving and faithful wife. You have never taken lightly our marriage vows:

"In sickness and in health, to love and to cherish, as long as we both shall live."

Special Thanks To:

The Canadian Cancer Society for their vigilant care of cancer patients and promotion of research to find a cure for this dreaded disease.

The London Regional Cancer Program at the London Health Sciences Centre, Victoria Hospital, London, Ontario, for administering help to the helpless and hope to the hopeless.

My medical team—including all the doctors, nurses, and staff—who have touched my life, both past and present.

Our family and friends who have supported us with their encouragement and prayers.

My wife, Sharon, for her loving care throughout the good and the not-so-good times, and for her assistance in editing this manuscript.

The staff of Word Alive Press for guiding me in the publishing of this book.

Table of Contents

Initial Perspective

Retirement crept up on me way too fast. Health issues were the culprit. Mark Twain said, "Life would be infinitely happier if we could only be born at the age of eighty and gradually approach eighteen" (*Autobiography with Letters*, William L. Phelps). Someone else said, "Don't let aging get you down. It's too hard to get back up!"

Well, I'm neither down nor out, even after coming through five bouts of cancer: thyroid, skin, lung, prostate, and kidney. Today I feel amazingly healthy. The thyroid and lung cancers are gone. Skin cancer is in remission, and the prostate and kidney cancers are still within the five-year surveillance regimen but with hopeful outlook.

Let me give you some *perspective* on how this all came to pass.

When I was eight, lumps had formed in my neck. For three years, they were observed and biopsied and finally diagnosed as malignant. Surgery removed the larger tumors and most of my thyroid, and cobalt radiation treatments followed. For me it was an adventure. For my parents—a nightmare! Years later, my mom told me how our church had prayed for me around the clock the night before, and the day of, my surgery.

At my tenth-year checkup, Doctor F. told me I no longer needed to worry about thyroid cancer. "If you ever get cancer again," he assured me, "it will have no connection to this."

Turning his attention away from my chart, he gently changed the subject. "So what are you studying in college?"

"Music."

"And what's your major?"

"Singing."

"You're kidding!" he responded. "That's amazing. The cobalt radiation was applied so close to your vocal cords we were concerned whether you would even be able to speak."

Perspective was born in my heart that day. Not only had my life been spared—so had my voice. From that moment on, I knew that my decision to serve the Lord with my gift in music was the right career choice. Since God had preserved my voice, I could do no less than use it for His glory and in ministry to His church.

In my early forties, skin cancer showed up. One day when my dermatologist, Dr. A., was surgically removing a larger basil cell, I nonchalantly commented. "Skin cancer isn't really life threatening, is it, Doctor?"

"It certainly can be," she sternly replied. "Especially if you don't diligently do what you're told and follow every precaution I have suggested."

My lung cancer was discovered in 2004. I have never smoked. Yet this cancer was similar to a smoker's cancer and considered very aggressive. That journey inspired my book, *Musing and Muttering through Cancer.*

At my five-year checkup, the oncologist entered the exam room with a huge smile on his face. "In all my years of experience," he declared, "I have only told this to a handful of people. Your lung cancer is gone."

Again my *perspective* was re-focused. I realized more than ever how precious life is.

Checkups are like Forrest Gump's box of chocolates. *You never know what you're going to get!* For over ten years, I had undergone routine prostate checkups including several biopsies, all of which had come back benign. Then, in

2009, I was asked to be part of a test group at the Robarts Research Institute in London, Ontario.

Utilizing a new biopsy technique, which produced a three dimensional image, the radiologists discovered cancer already outside the prostate capsule. Surgery was scheduled followed by radiation. The result was encouraging.

However, during the third follow-up visit with my urologist, the CT scan showed tumors on both my kidneys. These tumors were burned out with a relatively new medical procedure called radio frequency ablation. Some of the chapters in this book make reference to both the prostate and kidney cancer experiences.

From my limited *perspective*, God is not finished with me yet. No, he is not punishing me; he is teaching me. Obviously, I am a slow learner! But I am not bothered by the process. I'm content. Honestly, I want God's agenda to be my agenda. If I live, I live. If I die, I go to be with the Lord Jesus in heaven. It's a win-win scenario.

The words *"gaining perspective"* describe how I am a work in progress. Each story and poem illustrates how my view of life is being shaped. I'm realizing more than ever that God is at work in me and in all the experiences I face. His presence is for real.

I hope you are helped in your journey through reading this. Perhaps through gaining insight into my perspective on life and faith, yours might be influenced in a positive way as well. I also hope you gain new personal *perspective* on the mercy and grace of our Lord Jesus Christ and His love for you.

Doing or Being?

September 2007

For most of my life, music ministry defined who I was—music teacher, music missionary, music pastor, music director, music, music, music. Doing defined my being. It is not a good thing when one's profession defines one's person. That happens when what we do becomes more significant than who we are. When all the doing is done, the being can become a real drag.

Looking back, I realize that many people were impacted in a positive way through what I did. My students went on to make their own impact. Indigenous and Spanish churches in Ecuador, where we were missionaries in the late 1970s and early 1980s, were helped in their emerging praise and worship. Churches where I served in Canada were influenced to mature in worship and be more tolerant of one another's preferred styles. Concerts attracted many people from outside the church, opening new horizons of faith.

But I have to admit that as I approach official retirement without a full-time music ministry, life feels rather empty. I entered what felt like a downward slope in 2005 when I underwent chemotherapy for lung cancer. For the next two years, my ministry was limited to being a part-time volunteer in music and worship in the same church where, prior to my cancer, I had been pastor of Worship Ministries. It felt strange having a workload reduced to fifteen hours a week. My heart wanted to carry the responsibility of the former full-time load, but my body could only manage a portion of it. During those two years, I was forced to realize the unlikelihood of ever returning to full-time ministry. When my volunteer work began to lead to more stress than was good for me, we decided to move to London, Ontario, closer to family.

So what am I going to do now? You see? There it is again—*do*.

Early retirement, I'm discovering, has some significant advantages. It's great to be able to visit many family members who now live only an hour or so away. There has been the "settling-in" process. No end, it seems, to putting everything in place and turning a condo into our home. But when it's all done, then what?

It's true that we all need something to do. You just can't sit and stare at a wall—or TV! Visiting family and friends will be much more frequent, for sure. Finding and settling into a local church is an ongoing process as well. Discovering a venue for volunteering somewhere is a targeted ingredient in this new life, as is reading, writing, and hopefully a little golf.

The most significant questions are "Who am I? What am I? What have I become?"

Hopefully I have moved on from basing my self-worth on my profession. My focus now is to develop meaningful tasks that grow out of who I am. One thing is for sure. I am committed to following Jesus Christ. I am what I am by His grace. Being committed to Him, I know that I am forgiven. I am a child of God. And I am available to do whatever He wants me to do. I also need to be who He wants me to be.

Jesus says, "I am the vine; you are the branches. If you remain in me and I in you, you will bear much fruit; apart from me you can do nothing" (John 15:5).

LIFE

Life, so full of pressures and demands,
  you have a crafty way
    of pressuring the one in whom you dwell.
For quite some time I was a slave
  to you and to your constant prod:
    "Go here. Go there.
      Do this. Do that."
It all seemed more and more a bore
  until I talked to God.
You see, 'midst all the duties of each day,
  although they all were good,
    they usually were rather necessary too.
Yet still there was a lack.
There was no room
  to meditate upon such basic things
    as why go here,
      or why do that?
Nor was there time to contemplate
  the goodness of the Lord.
Subsequently that which I was doing
  had an empty sound.
No ring of joy.
  No resonance of love,
    until I talked to God.
I found that life itself is just like that,
  unless it centers in the One
    who gives *abundant life*.

Shining Bright!

November 2007

Nicely settled in London since August, and thankful to God for His guidance and provision, we are already looking forward to the Christmas season! But this year is very different. Rather than directing a Christmas production, I'm singing in one. It feels very different being on the opposite side of the podium. I am patiently resisting moments of inclination to make suggestions or to put my oar in. I guess its all part of getting used to retirement.

Having retired in June, and unlike most years in church music ministry, I didn't have to spend the summer months choosing Christmas music in order for it to arrive in time for the first rehearsal in September. No more hectic fall months either, rehearsing for Sunday services and Christmas concerts.

On November 7, 2007, Sharon and I were suddenly transported back one year in our memories. We received an e-mail from our friend, Norbert Kondraki, who had been our drama director for last year's concert. Before sharing the story he passed on to us, here is a bit of background.

In preparation for the 2006 concert, our pastor had mentioned that he thought the topic of "Light" would be very appropriate. It would tie in with the direction of the overall ministry of the season. This was my fourth year directing "The Living Christmas Tree" concert series at First Baptist

Church—a Millennium project for the city of Orillia. We presented the concert five times on the weekend before Christmas with attendance totalling around three thousand people. The thirty-five-foot tree held seventy choir members. Several thousand lights on it, controlled by computer, gave a variety of effects as needed in the various songs. The concerts were very definitely light-driven.

Sometimes, the simplest little things create moments of greatest impact. Sharon came up with the idea of handing out little key fob lights to all the audience to be turned on during "Silent Night." The entire auditorium would be darkened and everyone would let their tiny light shine. The key fobs were incredibly effective as everyone contributed to a brilliant blue midnight effect as they quietly sang, "Silent night, holy night, all is calm, all is bright."

For months afterward, people were still excited about these little lights, using them in all kinds of situations. We encouraged people to keep it handy, using it as a key ring, and be reminded of its inscription: "Light your world."

Now, here is the story from Norbert:

Last week, my wife, Margaret, met a woman at the Lighthouse here in Orillia who told her about an incident involving her husband. The woman was someone who happened to be working at the Lighthouse that day. Sometime in the summer, her husband and a younger man were out boating on Georgian Bay and got caught in a storm. Unfortunately, they soon were in trouble as their boat capsized. In the meantime, the family became concerned and then worried when the two did not return. A rescue team was called in from Trenton and a search began. Throughout the night, the search team found nothing.

Then, in the early morning hours, a search plane scouting the coast line happened to catch sight of a small but bright pin of light cutting into the pre-dawn darkness. Sure enough, the light was emanating near the two lost men. The two men had drifted to shore holding on to the boat and both collapsed on the shoreline. On finding the two men, they discovered that the light was from a small key fob hanging from the belt of the older man. It somehow shorted and stayed in the "on" position. The fob was given to this man last Christmas, in Orillia, at "The Living Christmas Tree" concert. I pray that this fob saved not only his physical life.

You see, David, how you touched people?

(Used with permission from Norbert Kondraki)

We were thrilled to hear this story and realize that these men were indeed helped. We have heard of many folk who were impacted with our Christmas concerts in the past. It wasn't because of us. It was a group effort, and the final results were always a "God thing."

Though we are not presently preoccupied with planning concerts, as we were in the past, opportunities to participate in the glorious music of Christmas are bound to arise each year. No doubt, when they do, we will be reminded of the good old days that are sometimes only as good as our bad old memories!

Breakfast with Mr. Grey

January 2008

There is nothing quite like a bowl of hot oatmeal for breakfast. That's our routine, not that I am so thrilled about eating oatmeal every day. Notice that I said "nothing." I lied; I would actually prefer bacon and eggs! But over the past several years, Sharon has helped me to become more aware of what I should and should not indulge in. She, having to keep close tabs on her own cholesterol count, and I, needing to keep close tabs on my pound count, agree on many matters pertaining to diet. If we were totally consistent, we would abstain from snacks later in the day. Then I could write a diet book and call it "How Oatmeal Changed My Size!"

This morning, I began my same-old-same-old breakfast of a bowl of oatmeal and a glass of orange juice, followed by half a toasted bagel with jam, and a cup of coffee. I said grace, thanking the Lord with the same-old-same-old prayer He hears day after day.

As I looked up from my brief prayer, there in the bird feeder was a pudgy grey squirrel filling his face with birdseed. I don't imagine he's trying to grow wings or feathers. He just seems to like eating birdseed. I mean, if I were in the business of feeding squirrels the feeder would look much different. For one thing, it would have a much wider platform for him to sit on. As it is, he balances precariously on a little ledge built for sparrows. But there he was, eating nonstop hand to mouth, packing it away cheek to cheek for future fare.

That's okay. Wise Solomon once said, "The godly care for their animals, but the wicked are always cruel" (Proverbs 12:10, NLT). I would rather be the former.

Commenting on how London squirrels seem to be predominantly grey, unlike the black and red squirrels at our former Bolsover home, we carried on our leisurely breakfast giving him little attention. Sharon and I then prayed together (our custom after breakfast), remembering the needs of many of our friends and family members who are going through tough times. Then as I'm sure most loving, retired husbands do, I cleaned up the kitchen while Sharon did other more important things.

Funny thing was, after I finished the dishes, there was Mr. Grey still filling his face with birdseed. How can such a little animal eat for so long? At least I assume he was eating. Being all stooped over, as he was, maybe he was engaged in his own prayer time.

Do animals and birds pray? I really never thought about it much. One thing I do know is that they don't worry about stuff near as much as we do. They have a more Faithful Feeder than I will ever be. Referring to our Creator God, the Psalmist says:

"Even the wild animals cry out to you because the streams have dried up, and fire has consumed the wilderness pastures" (Joel 1:20, NLT).

"He gives food to the wild animals...when they cry" (Psalm 147:9, NLT).

So obviously God hears their cry, whether it is from bowed heads or empty tummies. But here is something even more amazing. Mr. Grey expresses praise to God along with the whole world. It's true. Reading the following Psalm selection causes me to ask why I'm so skimpy in my praise to God for a bowl of hot oatmeal:

> Praise the LORD from the earth, you creatures of the ocean depths, fire and hail, snow and clouds, wind and weather that obey him, mountains and all hills, fruit trees and all cedars, wild animals and all livestock, small scurrying animals and birds, kings of the earth and all people, rulers and judges of the earth, young men and young women, old men and children. Let them all praise the name of the LORD. For his name is very great; his glory towers over the earth and heaven!
>
> Psalm 148:7–13 (NLT)

Precious Moments

March 2008

C rash! So much for that ceramic plate! It's a wonder that everyone in our condo block didn't wake up. Sharon surely did.

Trying not to sound traumatized, my laryngitic voice squeaked, "I'm okay. I just knocked something off the wall."

It happened in the middle of the night. Actually it was closer to morning because I had already been up twice gargling with salt water, desperately trying to clear my congested throat. The two Saturday evening Easter concerts had gone well. Three more were only hours away starting at 9:00 a.m. I had sustained just enough voice and energy to make it through the vocally demanding songs, in spite of a tessitura laced with extremely high tenor notes.

In the past, I had no difficulty with a range like that. But the doctors at the voice clinic in Vancouver, who checked me over about a decade ago, are proving to be right. They said that the radiation I received as a child for thyroid cancer had left scar tissue on my vocal chords. They said, "You've managed to sing over it or through it in your younger days, but it will give you more and more trouble as you grow older."

No doubt about it. One day I have a clear voice. The next, I sound like a foghorn and my range is significantly diminished—especially if I have sung high and loud too long.

So there I stood by the sink in the middle of the night wishing I had not overused my delicate vocal cords and hoping to preserve enough for three more concerts. As I reached for a tissue, my hand knocked a ceramic plate off its holder, and it smashed into pieces on the floor, doomed to the fate of Humpty-Dumpty. I hadn't looked at this plate for years. It was just there making the wall look nice. But as I picked up the pieces, I noticed that it was a *"Precious Moments"* plate—you know, the ones with the pretty, little, soft pastel people. This one had a music theme. It was titled, "Let Heaven and Nature Sing." On it was inscribed a certification number: #2943 of a Christmas Collection dated 1982. Ironically, it was a gift from one of my vocal students of yesteryear.

"Precious Moments! Yeah, right. I could use one about now!" I moaned to myself.

I finally drifted off to sleep for another hour only to be awakened by the alarm clock. Time to get up, gargle some more, and try to get the voice going again. As I opened my mouth to sing a couple of notes, nothing came out. Then, with a little coaxing of the vocal apparatus, I managed a wee croak. For an hour I lightly vocalized wishing I could sing bass instead of tenor!

In John 16:23–24, Jesus says, "Very truly I tell you, my father will give you whatever you ask in my name... ask and you will receive, and your joy will be complete."

I don't always presume that my will has to be God's will, but in this case, I made a very specific request. "Lord, if you want me to sing today, I need a voice."

He had done it often before. Why would I doubt Him now?

It was time to head over to the church. I kept humming lightly, wondering, *Is God going to come through again? Because if he doesn't, I'm in deep trouble.*

I forgot to mention that not only do I sing in the choir, but I had been given the responsibility of being section leader as well. Each of the section leaders is given a microphone, allowing the sound operator to balance the choir over the musical instruments.

"Lovely! Where can I hide?" Anxiety was definitely setting in.

It seemed no time till we were starting. As soon as we began the first song, I knew God had done it again. Talk about *Precious Moments*!

Humpty-Dumpty may be irreparable, but not me. As long as God gives me a voice to sing, I'll sing. That's been true my whole life. Nothing has changed—except my scary vocal cords. That's "scary," with scars—not "scary, "spooky!

My singing is probably already on borrowed time. But for now, yet again, my joy is complete.

So What of Excellence?

When excellence is found, a price was paid.
Not always with cold cash, but costly just the same.
The price of excellence reflects an effort and a skill
that's fashioned over time;
tempered by the heat of raw experience.

Sometimes I feel coerced to mediocrity.
How sickening and abhorrent,
offering a pittance of my time
to fill a lazy role.
Or frittering away the talent given by God
requiring years to hone.

Should meaningless routine be kept alive
while shirking creativity and work?
Why let potential beauty go to pot,
and excellence be slain
upon the altar of the easy way;
the seemingly more enjoyable,
and less demanding way?
No sweat, nor tears, nor aches or pains.
A modest cost, but not enough to hurt!

So does it really matter much,
that one would stand in awe,
amazed at excellence,
relieved that mediocrity
has once again been bruised?

Oh yes it does!
It matters greatly what they think, and more.
It matters to the Lord,
the God of excellence, the Mighty One,
Creator of all things,
the God who said that it was good
each time.

So what of excellence?
May I today take special care
to rise above mere basic expectations,
and offer to the Lord a sacrifice of praise.

© 1993, David Gast

Four-Leaf Clovers

June 2008

This morning's walk was spectacular. The rain had stopped, and as I stepped out onto the street and made my way to the river path, tepid air filled my nostrils with the sweet scent of spring. The pathway meanders along the bank of the Upper Thames River, through a dense forest, out into a small meadow, back into more forest and over a picturesque bridge that I remembered had been totally submerged during our recent floods.

The morning song of a plethora of birds, warbling and twittering louder than usual, filled the air around me. Each call was unique, distinct in itself. Yet all were blended into a melodious symphony. *What robust songs of praise to God*, I thought to myself, *coming from these tiny creatures that have been so silent during the past few stormy days!*

A young lady was standing on the bridge, facing the river, with head bowed and hands clasped below her chin. I stopped and quietly watched for a moment, realizing that she too, like the birds, could be lifting her soul to the Lord. Suddenly I realized that my gawking could be misunderstood! So I walked a few yards farther to the patch of clover that had caught my eye only a week ago and where I had found some four-leaf clovers and a five-leaf clover as well!

Finding four, five, and sometimes six-leaf clovers has been a passion for me. I can't walk by clover anywhere without looking down to see if one stands out. In case you're wondering, I have very little Irish blood in my veins! When I was a child, my aunt Doris, when visiting our farm, would sit on the lawn and find them with very little effort. Intrigued, I began to have an eye for them myself. One day I discovered a four-leaf clover patch near our horse barn, similar to the one I have described.

Kneeling down, still with the image of the lady on my mind, I picked seven clovers quite quickly and saw several others. Those I left untouched, thinking that perhaps someone else would like to experience the joy of discovery.

Then an idea came to mind. I turned to see if the young lady was still there. She was gone. Too bad. It would have been nice to have given her one. I could have said something like, "Here's a four-leaf clover for you. This is not a lucky charm but rather a tiny unique piece of God's creation. It's as unique as every one of those birds singing to Him in the trees. This can be a reminder to you that you too are unique and special to God."

Could've, would've, should've—always disappointing. Daydreaming done, I completed my walk, carefully bringing my four-leaf treasures home to be refreshed in a vase of cool water.

Sauntering back to the computer room, I noticed the answering machine was blinking. There was only one message—from my brother, Roger, with more news about my mother's progress.

A week and a half ago, she broke her hip. It was a bad break. She underwent surgery in spite of a very high level of risk that she might not pull through. However, she did. But yesterday an x-ray indicated that the plate had pulled away from the bone, leaving her in ongoing agonizing pain. Roger's news from the surgeon was that she is confident Mom can tolerate a second surgery. They would put a pin down through the center of the bone for greater stability. That's scheduled for Thursday.

She doesn't need our good thoughts or the luck of the Irish. She needs our prayers. No, my four-leaf clovers are not lucky charms. They have no special powers. But I know Someone who does. This morning, before breakfast, I read this: "But I trust in you, Lord. I say, 'You are my God.' My times are in your hands" (Psalm 31:14–15a).

So are Mom's, and so are mine. Yours are as well.

Broken Windows

July 2008

Thwack! I heard it all the way from the front room. What in the world was that?

"Dave, come quickly," Sharon's cry of panic got my immediate attention.

Carefully dismounting the ladder I was on, I laid down my paintbrush and ran to the bedroom. Sharon was pale with fear as she pointed to the bay window. It was smashed. Both panes were still intact but cracked side to side and top to bottom with a two-inch hole in the outer pane. The inner one was broken but still held together.

Sharon had been sitting at her desk located right in front of that window. The fellows, contracted by our condo group, were mowing our tiny yard—one of the blessings of condo living. But this time it turned out to be less than a blessing. Zooming round and about, his riding mower had hit the top of a water main, sending pieces of cast iron flying through the air. Fortunately, or rather by the mercy of God, Sharon's life was spared. Thank God that that piece of metal didn't penetrate both panes of the window.

How quickly our lives can be altered! How fragile our security apart from the grace of God. Yet how life often drags on and on, day in and day out, with little change! No sudden surprises. No thwacks to jolt us into reality.

I am reminded of that with the slow passing of my mother. It was seven weeks ago she fell and broke her hip.

From that moment on and through two surgeries the following week, she has existed with very little sustenance. She is drugged heavily with morphine to control the intense pain. Not only has she suffered from her broken hip, but also with advanced osteoporosis and a deep and dangerous bedsore that started weeks ago in the hospital.

She has been literally wasting away for over a month now. The nurses and staff have given her the best of care, way beyond our expectations. We love every one of them and are truly amazed at how they love and care for Mom. Four times since June 19 we have been called to come, for they were sure she had only hours left. Then to all of our amazement, she rallied again, only to face more anxiety and pain and weakness, yearning deeply to go to be with the Lord in heaven.

Today I have stayed at home. Roger, who lives nearby, will be dropping in several times again today to see how she is, just as he has been doing continually throughout the ordeal.

For Mom's sake, we've gotten to the place of longing that God would just take her. If He would reach down and gather her gently into His loving arms—soon, quickly. Thwack. No more pain. No more suffering. If only it were that easy. But are we ready for the impact it will have on us—the pain, the loss?

As we have gazed into the window of her life, family times have been extra special, cherishing special memories and reliving treasured experiences of life with Mom. But her window will soon be shut. Waiting, watching, we squint with blurry eyes through cracks created by the impact of her imminent death.

The shattered pane in our bedroom will be fixed very soon. But the thwack of Mom's departure will require time to heal. Broken hearts mend slowly. But God comforts the broken-hearted, as should we:

> Praise be to the God and Father of our Lord Jesus Christ, the Father of compassion and the God of all comfort, who comforts us in all our troubles, so that we can comfort those in any trouble with the comfort we ourselves receive from God.
>
> 2 Corinthians 1:3–4

See there? God isn't into thwacking. He knows what is best for Mom, for us as a family, and for you.

Get It Right!

August 2008

So who's perfect? Anyone want to step up to the plate? Have you noticed that batting 500 is really good? Batting 1,000 just never happens. Ty Cobb (professional baseball player from 1905–1928) still holds the top career batting average at 366. One can't be thrown off by, "He swings—he misses." It's expected.

So why do I get my shirt in a knot whenever I mess up? Just when I try to get it right, something goes wrong. People say, "Oh, that's okay. Don't worry about it. We all make mistakes. None of us is perfect."

True. But…

On Friday, July 25, 2008, we celebrated the life and faith of my mother, Jean Gast. She went to be with her Lord and Saviour on July 22. For weeks we had anticipated her departure, watching her struggle with pain and discomfort. During that rollercoaster ride, I had compiled a funeral service based on data that Mom had meticulously left for us. The service outline and a synopsis of her life were printed in a lovely folded bulletin with her picture on the front.

The day arrived. Everything was ready. I picked up the bulletins from the printer, and the first thing that caught my eye was the picture. It was okay, but the colour was a little off. I wanted so much to get it right. But I had not asked to see a proof before running off two hundred. That was mistake number one. My inner voice was saying, "You didn't get it right."

Mom's funeral was phenomenal. Uplifting. At visitation, the night before, there had been a steady stream of friends and family. It was like a four-hour hug. Next day the funeral went without a hitch. Everyone who took part excelled themselves.

Pastor Roy Lawson challenged us with a great sermon from the Gospel of John, chapter 12, about Mary who "did what she could, did all she could, and did it while she could." He noted that Mom was just like Mary. Pastor Roy got it right!

Grandson Josh gave a wonderful eulogy. He got it right!

My brother Karl gave a tribute that came straight from his heart. He sure got it right!

I even sang a solo and didn't break down.

My older brother Roger gave a tribute to Mom's faith on behalf of us three sons. He also officiated at the burial service and did it well. He, too, got it right.

Mom was truly honoured and would have been so thrilled because she also had a streak of perfectionism in her. She loved to get it right.

Two days later, reality suddenly struck. As I lay in a hot bath of Epsom salts trying to ease an aching back and sciatica, Sharon's urgent voice broke the stillness. "Oh, no! There is a terrible error on Mom's bulletin."

"A what?" I retorted.

"The date of Mom's death is incorrect!"

I couldn't believe it. I thought I had been so careful. She was right. It said March 22, 2008, instead of July 22. How could it have happened? We can't even call it a "chemo moment," which has become my standard excuse for imperfection. I just plain didn't get it right.

I realize now it doesn't really matter in the big scheme of things. But the next time I try writing something important, I will be sure to have Sharon edit it!

Recently I was reading Proverbs 31:25–31 relating the verses to my mom and to Sharon. Wow, this is special!

She is clothed with strength and dignity;
>   she can laugh at the days to come.
She speaks with wisdom,
>   and faithful instruction is on her tongue.
She watches over the affairs of her household
>   and does not eat the bread of idleness.
Her children arise and call her blessed;
>   her husband also, and he praises her:
"Many women do noble things,
>   but you surpass them all."
Charm is deceptive, and beauty is fleeting;
>   but a woman who fears the LORD is to be praised.
Honor her for all that her hands have done,
>   and let her works bring her praise at the city gate.

Just Another Holiday

October 2008

Years ago when I was young and our son Marty was much younger, his rock band, Emit Ridge, wrote a song titled "Holiday." The song says that after celebrating Christ's birthday, festivities over, decorations packed away, and everything has returned to normal, all they'll say is that it was "just another holiday."

Though it is somewhat satirical in its thrust, I understand clearly what they were getting at. Christmas is so heavily steeped in tradition and routine that we diminish its real significance with an ever-escalating preoccupation with ourselves and an insatiable appetite for stuff and merriment.

As I write this, we have just finished our Thanksgiving Celebration. Did we celebrate Thanksgiving well? We ate a lot! We laughed a lot. We also enjoyed playing Wii games—bowling especially and tennis. And I suppose baseball. Well, not so much baseball. Seems no one could hit the ball!

Several of us went for a long walk beside the Thames River to wear off some turkey. The weather was perfect. The foliage was stunning in its developing beauty, even on the sycamore trees. (Few people know that sycamore trees grow naturally in Southern Ontario; I only recently discovered that fact with the help of the Internet.)

Yes, we celebrated Thanksgiving well, at least in the traditional way. But our few verbal tokens of gratitude around the table hadn't happened as I had anticipated. We each contributed something that we were thankful for, but it quickly disintegrated into silliness. I didn't mind though because it was fun to hear everyone bantering back and forth. As grace was said before the meal, we thanked God for the gift of His Son and thanked Him that our security is in Christ our Lord and not in the struggling economy or the plummeting stock market.

Now, for the next big event—Christmas! It has become almost unmanageable. Retailers depend on it for the year's largest intake. Companies can go belly-up if sales drop by only a small percentage. We all fall into routine, like Canada geese flying south. Just take a few moments and watch the shoppers in follow-the-leader formation, honking for position, getting into long lineups with frustration and determination written all over their faces.

Many folk, just like those Canada geese, do fly south. We call them snowbirds. But don't snowbirds actually arrive in Canada just in time for the snow? I thought they were the flocks of little white birds flitting here and there over the snowbanks. In spite of this misnomer, our Canadian snowbirds leave in order to *miss* the snow. It's just the thing to do, especially if you are retired.

"Besides," they reason, "we have been doing this for years. Who wants to face snow and ice when you can walk on warm sandy beaches in your bare feet?"

Good point.

Some snowbirds wait to go south until Christmas celebrations are over. I wonder why. It's just another holiday, isn't it? Or is it? Perhaps being with family is an essential part of the celebration. However, the biblical account leaves us a bit confused about that. Mary and Joseph left their home and travelled to Joseph's hometown to pay taxes. Jesus left His Father and came to live with us. It was not just another holiday and meaningless routine. The smelly stable was hardly conducive to enjoying Christmas pudding.

Central to the whole event was giving and helping the needy. God gave. The innkeeper gave. Mary and Joseph were on the receiving end, and so are we. The old cliché, *Jesus is the Reason for the Season*, remains. We would all do well to spend more energy thinking and talking about that than worrying about preparations for "just another holiday."

Holiday

You threw a party for the world
Everyone was there
Tuxedo attitude
Plenty of nothing to share
Stand and laugh and look with me
Beside the artificial tree
Join the carols of the choir
The truth sings quietly

The room is quiet now again
The decorations fall
Out come the attic box and barrels
To snatch them all, all again
Keep it, hide it all away
For just another holiday
Keep it, hide it all away
For just another holiday

Ribbons, ties and fancy suits
Shallow smiles and empty handshakes

Will someone tell them of the story
The season quickly awakes
Today sleeps the season
And the world falls back to place
Will you wake me up
The next time Christ has a birthday?

That's all they'll say
Just another holiday
That's all they'll say
Just another holiday

But you kept one tree alive
Bare, without a temperate glow
Except the brightest star you left with me
I met a man behind a different tree.
Twelve times a thousand times a restoration
The joy of that first day
Twelve times a thousand times a restoration
The joy of that first day

And it's not just another holiday
It's not just another holiday

©1991, Marty Gast and Emit Ridge
Used with permission.

On the Ice

January 2009

I went skating this morning. The last time I was on skates was eight years ago, but it seems like a century ago. Skating has not been part of my life for a long time. And the sad thing is that I used to love skating. In younger years, a winter wouldn't go by without me being on the ice regularly.

A few weeks ago, I put our skates in the trunk of the car thinking we might share some ice time with our granddaughters in Waterloo. It never happened. But this morning, after letting Sharon off at work, I got this radical idea to drop by the outdoor ice rink at Victoria Park. The radio weather reports indicated that the temperature had warmed up to minus twelve degrees, but there was a wind chill of minus twenty. That's okay. I'm pretty tough. So as I arrived, much to my delight, the rink was totally empty. That was a relief as I imagined what I might look like getting on to the ice.

For some dumb reason, instead of going into the dressing room, I decided to don my skates on one of the nearby park benches. Brushing the snow aside, I uncovered a butt-freezing area and sat down. First, I had to untie the knot that had bound my skates together for the past eight years. Off came my gloves, and my fingers immediately complained, "What are you doing?"

I didn't respond. I think my brain was a bit frozen too because I took off my right boot way too soon. The skate

30

was so cold and stiff, it took forever to pry it open and get my foot in. Already my fingers felt like popsicles, making it almost impossible to tighten the laces.

Finally—one skate on and one to go! I started stuffing my fingers in my mouth, blowing hot air on them. That didn't help much, so with great haste and dogged determination, on went the second skate, albeit a little bit loose, and I hobbled shakily to the edge of the ice.

It's a scary moment when, all by yourself, you step onto a slick ice surface having not done so for umpteen years. But gingerly I took the step, wobbled a bit, and glided off to a great start. Then the thought dawned on me; if Sharon only knew, she would be worrying that I would break my neck or have a heart attack or concussion or worse.

Not to worry! I discovered that skating seemed as natural as it ever did. I glided round and round turning one way and then the other. I even tried skating backward a bit until I realized that my skates were way too loose. Back to the bench I went for a tightening. By now my fingers had no more complaints. They were either dead or had gone into hibernation for the rest of the winter. After getting the laces all tightened up, I skated energetically round and round, frontward and backward until I knew that the parking meter time was about to expire.

It was exhilarating! And during that half hour, I found myself thinking a lot about my dad. At his funeral, just a few days ago, it was mentioned that in his young adult life he used to be the best skater around. I miss Dad and all his words of wisdom.

Dad said that skating is like riding a bicycle. You never forget how. He was right. When he first took me to the rink as a child, I more or less walked on my skates. He told me I had to push off on one foot and glide, then push off on the other, and so on and not to look down and not to try going too fast. "If you look down, you'll fall down. Push off, glide. Push off, glide."

Our faith is similar, don't you think? The Bible says, "For we walk by faith, not by sight" (2 Corinthians 5:7, KJV). Walking requires one step at a time. Faith requires trusting God one step at a time. We need to keep our eyes on the Lord and in His word. If we look down, we'll slip and fall. The Bible also says, "Let us run with patience" (Hebrews 12:1, KJV). That means get moving, but don't be in a hurry. There's nothing there about skating, but it does say, "Those who hope in the LORD will renew their strength. They will soar on wings like eagles" (Isaiah 40:31).

Push off, glide. Push off, glide.

Next time I'm on the ice, maybe I should try some fancy figures. Then again, maybe I should stick to the basics Dad taught me—both on and off the ice.

I Cried Today

February 2009

I had a good cry this morning. You know, the kind that leaves you feeling relieved. They say tears can be cleansing. It's true. Dad's death on January 23 was not unexpected. He had been noticeably failing since Mom died in July. But all of a sudden, we realized that he was not going to live to be a hundred, but possibly leave us at ninety-five. And so he did.

That day, I had left his room for only about fifteen minutes, and when I returned, he had already passed into the arms of Jesus. I was stunned. A feeling of loneliness swept over me. I may have shed a tear, but I didn't cry. A sense of peace gripped my heart as I contemplated his being with our Lord.

But this morning, close to two weeks later, I had a good cry. I had decided to visit the gravesite which is only a short distance from our home. As I drove into Forest Lawn Cemetery, there was not a soul visible. I guess souls aren't visible anyway. Or are they? But you get the picture. I was alone.

After parking near the gravesite, I trudged through the snowbanks that had gathered since the day of the burial. As I arrived, the stark reality of death overwhelmed me. I just stood there, quiet. Gentle flurries were falling on the frozen floral arrangement placed there following the burial. There I stood.

As my thoughts began to focus on the reality and finality of death, I began talking to my dear departed father. Expressions of thanksgiving spilled out one after another:

Thank you, Dad, for being such a great example to me. Thank you for providing for our family and for being such a loving and supportive husband to our dear mother. Thank you for teaching me to work hard and to finish the job. Thank you for encouraging me to follow my dreams. Thank you for your steadiness and faith in God in the midst of incredible trials and losses. That faith was always clearly evident. Never once did I hear you curse or swear. Never once did I doubt your commitment to Christ.

And, Mom, thank you for being a wonderful mother. Thank you for your contagious smile and winsome personality. Thank you for your stern discipline, always administered wisely. It became clear, with the passing of time, that love for us was always your motivation. Thank you for loving each of us sons. I never ever doubted that love. Thank you for patiently enduring my reluctant piano practicing, and for believing in me, encouraging me to be my best. Thank you for praising God in the midst of the difficulties and trials of your life and for your consistent walk with the Lord.

My quiet thoughts and audible words turned into a prayer to my heavenly Father. It seemed natural to break into song, and I found myself singing the song my brother, Karl, sang at Dad's funeral. "My Jesus I love Thee, I know Thou art mine." When I got to "I'll love Thee in life, I will love

Thee in death, and praise Thee as long as Thou lendest me breath," I began to sob. I cried. I wept. I mourned the loss of my dear parents. It was good.

"If ever I love Thee, my Jesus, 'tis now!" That love for Jesus was lived out by both Mom and Dad—daily, openly. Should I not do likewise without reservation?

TEARS

The tears of a heart of repentance
    wash clean the conscience of sin.
But tears of disobedience
    will never cleanse within.

The tears of the Saviour's followers
    were shed away from the cross.
They could not bear to be with Him.
    They could not face the cost.

The tears of Mary His mother
    fell hot on the burning sod,
beneath the cross of Jesus,
    the blameless Son of God.

The tears of we who nailed Him
    on Calvary's cruel tree
bring hope and true repentance,
    for all eternity.

© 1988 D. Gast, Ref. Luke 23:27–49

Here's Hoping

May 2009

Recently, I've been thinking about hope. It's a word I use all the time. You know the routine. Somebody is leaving on vacation, and we wish them well. "Hope you have a nice trip. Sure hope it doesn't rain. Hope there isn't a big lineup at the border. Hope you come back rested." It's all about the other person. The hope-er dishes out hope to the hope-ee, and really, that kind of hope has no substance at all. It's merely expressing our best wishes.

I suppose the thing that got me going on this is—well, two things actually. One is the results from a recent biopsy indicating that I have now joined the ranks of men with prostate cancer. A bone scan has indicated concern that migration may have taken place, so now I am scheduled for an x-ray and CT scan to investigate further. June 17 is when we are to find out. So like they say, "Here's hoping."

Actually, I *am* hoping. I'm *hoping in the Lord*. That leads me to the second thing that stimulated my thinking about hope—the many practical references to hope that I've been discovering in the Bible.

You may be thinking that *hoping in the Lord* sounds a bit overdone spiritually, but it's not meant to be. That was the way the apostle Paul expressed a practical decision he was making to send Timothy back to the church at Philippi. In Philippians 2:19 he said, "I hope in the Lord Jesus to send Timothy to you soon."

I like that because it welcomes Jesus into the nitty-gritty of life. He has been there with me all through my cancer journey. So acknowledging my need for His presence and help during these tests makes perfect sense. Ultimately, my hope is in the Lord. Whether the results are negative or positive (good or bad), I win if my hope is in Him. Psalm 16:8 says, "I keep my eyes always on the Lord. With him at my right hand, I will not be shaken." In other words, "I will not lose hope."

Losing hope is not a pretty picture because lost hope slams the door on the future. At least that's how it appears when hope is gone. There are countless people experiencing hopelessness as we speak. Life has spiralled downward with lost employment, lost health and lost purpose. Hope has vanished into the murky air of calamity and disappointment.

Where does one turn when hope is gone? The old saying, "pulling one's self up by the bootstraps," offers no help at all if you have lost your boots and the straps with them!

I just talked with the gardener who was working in front of our condo. He told me that he was laid off from the auto industry but has picked up this job, at least temporarily. Good for him! Some of you who read this may be in similar circumstances. Perhaps you can take steps to retrain, rebuild, or regroup. Maybe you can pour some creative juices into the mix and come up with a new direction or a new business or research the resources that are available through government and other agencies.

Not everyone needs employment insurance, but everyone needs God's assurance. Turning to Him in the middle of life's greatest crisis may be seen by some as a weakness. On the contrary, calling out to God in the midst of difficult times is positioning oneself in the strongest place possible.

Admitting we need His help is the best starting point for a new life. It brings hope alive. First Timothy 6:17 tells us to alert people not to "put their hope in wealth, which is so uncertain, but to put their hope in God, who richly provides us with everything for our enjoyment."

No wonder I'm hopeful!

Hope Is Alive
Sonnet

Strong flows the current of unending Hope;
Eternal heritage that rivals time.
Inheritance of faith, though weak in scope,
Is strong when anchored firm in Christ Divine.

When all is well and victories are won,
Why drag the days through doldrum drudgery?
What 'waits the weary, worried, wanting one
Who sits and sulks in silent misery?

A brighter day emerging, yet unseen,
Anticipates a better time ahead.
Though no one's ever promised life serene,
Hope is alive. Yes, Hope is never dead.

Our future lies not in our measured plans,
But rests securely in our Saviour's hands.

© 2008, David Gast

Trusting Again

June 2009

Trust me. This won't be the last time you hear from me! Here you are thinking, *Oh no. Not him again. Not another organ recital! We've already endured all his musings and mutterings through lung cancer."*

My last story indicated that I have now joined the ranks of men with prostate cancer. That discovery was followed by a CT scan and a bone scan. Initially, the bone scan indicated that perhaps the cancer had migrated, so it was followed up by a series of x-rays. Yesterday we met with Dr. C. Praise God, the mark on the eighth rib was of no concern, and they said there is no evidence of bone cancer. That's a big relief!

Knowing that the prostate cancer would have to be dealt with, we expected they would recommend surgery. We were right, and a prostatectomy is scheduled for September 4.

Dr. C. is known across Canada and beyond as a leader in the field of urology, having performed the first robotic laparoscopic prostatectomy in Canada. I don't qualify for that method because of the stage of my cancer. He told me he needs to go in with his hands in order to be as sure as possible to get it all. Depending on the outcome, I may require post-surgery radiation. I'm so grateful to have a trustworthy physician.

Speaking of trustworthy, who can you really trust these days? Politicians have us wondering. Economists have us confused. The media often seems biased. Advertisers and marketers are always telling me that my life is incomplete without their products. Besides that, I can't stand their high-pitch yelling on commercials. So who can I trust?

When it comes to our health, we are faced with unsettling statistics from renowned medical institutions that indicate survival percentages for surgeries, radiation treatments, chemotherapy, etc. Herbal and holistic methods by the dozen promise painless cures for every ailment. Dietary experts boast both prevention and cures. Everyone has an angle. Personally, I trust my medical team of doctors and specialists. Are they worthy of my trust? Yes, I believe they are—though not infallible.

But I know One who is incapable of making a mistake. In James 1:17 God is described as One "who does not change like shifting shadows." Psalm 9:10 tells me this: "Those who know your name trust in you, for you, LORD, have never forsaken those who seek you." Dr. C. also knows His name. He is a fine Christian surgeon who attends our church. Yes, I choose to put my trust in the Lord as I also trust my surgeon.

A number of months ago, we teamed up with some friends, Frank and Brenda Bale, to form a quartet that we have named *OASIS*, (an acronym for *Older Adults Sharing in Song*). We are booked for several seniors events in the fall. As it stands, my capability of concertizing can't be trusted—especially since the first event is scheduled the week following surgery! So we are praying for an earlier surgery date, which would uncomplicate things.

Oh well, part of trusting the Lord is learning to be flexible and content with limitations. I'm still a student in that area but eager to keep learning.

Yesterday I Was Shot

July 2009

You know the stress of getting ready for an exciting day. July 28, which seemed so far away a month ago, was suddenly here. I had packed the car the night before so that everything would be ready for an early departure. All I needed was a good sleep. But guess what? Sleep was hard to come by as I rehearsed over and over in my mind what the coming day would be like.

As I left the house, Sharon gave me a big hug and wished me well. Only one thing was left to do—pick up a few food items at the grocery store on the way. I was ready to face who-knows-what!

No, I wasn't going on a vacation. I wasn't going hunting or fishing or camping or golfing. The car was packed with props for the filming of *Choose Joy: Philippians in Person,* a dramatic monologue in which I present the book of Philippians. In costume, including chains, I portray the apostle Paul who wrote this letter while under house arrest in Rome. I have performed it on numerous occasions since memorizing it in 2003.

Upon arrival, I discovered the filming crew already setting up lights and camera equipment. At this point the stage was a mess. After briefly meeting a few of the crew members, I figured out where to set up my table of props, which include the gifts of Epaphroditus—part of the story. Everything was beginning to appear camera ready.

I'm thinking, *Am I up to this? Will I make a fool of myself—or worse yet, of the apostle Paul? Am I going to waste the time of all these professionals? Oh dear. Oh dear!*

It was time for my makeover. The director introduced me to the makeup person. She did an amazing job, starting by straightening my frizzy "chemo hair." Then she whitened it to make me look older. Finally, two and a half hours later, everything was ready: lighting, sound, monitoring equipment, makeup, costume, chains, and props. The time for filming had arrived.

It took no time for me to realize that the six crew members knew exactly what they were doing. But I wasn't confident that I did! About this time, my dear friend, Paul, quietly moved in beside me, put his hand on my shoulder, and said a prayer that only I and God could hear, finishing with, "And may this video be a blessing and inspiration to all who will see it as they see and hear the word of God."

It was time to focus now that I had everything in perspective.

"Rolling…Three, two, one, *action.*"

So this is what it feels like to get *shot*. Not bad, except when I forgot to act! That happened a few times. They were so patient with me. One of the lines in chapter four says: "Let your gentleness be evident to all." I saw gentleness demonstrated over and over by the crew. As the day progressed, I lost track of all the "takes" from this angle and that angle, close-ups, midrange shots and extra takes where I forgot important lines. Between them all was the ever-present Goldie diligently touching up my makeup and adjusting my costume.

Two things gripped me with increasing intensity throughout the day. First was my awareness of *the peace of God, guarding my heart and my mind.* It's in Philippians—i.e., my script. And it's true. My memory stayed intact, except for a few prompts here and there, and I was totally at peace.

The other gripping reality was the sciatic pain in my butt! We knew it was going to be an issue, and it was. But God gave me the strength and energy to persist. I experienced being able to "do all this through Him who gives me strength" (Philippians 4:13).

My desire was and is that this DVD of Philippians be "to the glory and praise of God" (Philippians 1:11). That was the whole point of the project. As he wrote this incredible letter while under house arrest in Rome, the Apostle Paul's desire was this: "That now as always, Christ will be exalted in my body, whether by life or by death" (Philippians 1:21).

As for the "life and death" part, I'm not sure I have fully arrived at the resolve Paul had. But even though I was shot yesterday, I'm still alive! The project is complete. The crew have gone home. And I am grateful, beyond words, to all who made it happen.

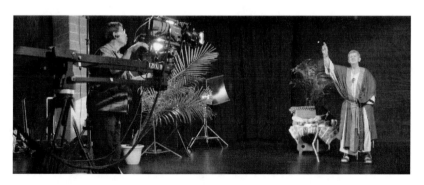

Philippians and Me

In early 2003, I was greatly inspired by two preteens who quoted from the sixth chapter of Romans in preparation for the pastor's sermon. Their presentation was dynamic—more than words and verses. The phrases came alive and were packed with emotion and meaning. I was impressed.

That week, challenged by what I had seen and heard, I began memorizing Philippians, which was where my daily readings happened to be. I already knew some verses from years gone by, and many others were very familiar, this being one of my favourite books of the Bible. Beginning at verse one, chapter one, I started what seemed to be a daunting task. Phrase by phrase, sentence by sentence, with countless repetitions I began to see results.

In about six months I had it completely memorized. Every time I went for a walk I would quote part or all of it. It takes only twenty-five minutes to recite all four chapters. The more I went over it, the clearer and more profound was its meaning. I began to understand, somewhat, the heart of the apostle Paul and the emotion with which he wrote this letter to the church at Philippi. I also began to sense that God had many things to say specifically to me. Little did I know that one year later I would be diagnosed with lung cancer. I was also unaware of how much Philippians would encourage and comfort me throughout that journey.

I presented it for the first time in our church on the last Sunday of 2003. Using one of the costumes from the Christmas pageant, a scroll representing Paul's letter, and some real chains for my ankles and wrists, I gave it my best shot. That was the first of many presentations I have given over the years.

Philippians is packed with truth that has given me a more positive perspective during these recent years. Here are some of the special things Philippians is teaching me:

- God isn't finished with me yet (1:6).
- Living is great as I invest my life in others (1:22).

- Dying is better by far because I will be with Christ in heaven (1:23).

- The struggles of life are an integral part of my faith in Christ (1:29).

- I need to be more humble and value others above myself (2:3).

- God is working in me to fulfill his good purpose for my life (2:12).

- Getting to know Christ may result in suffering (3:10–11).

- Knowing Christ brings assurance of life after death (3:10–11).

- Pressing on through life's challenges is worth every effort (3:12–14).

- My real home is in heaven. That's where I belong (3:20).

- I will have a new and transformed body in heaven (3:21).

- Instead of doubting, I need to stand firm in the Lord (4:1).

- Instead of worrying, I can pray and experience God's peace (4:6–7).

- It's better to focus on beautiful and positive things (4:8–9).

- Learning contentment isn't easy. We need God's help (4:11–13).

- God meets my scarcity with His abundance (4:19).

It All Depends

September 2009

Just two weeks before my prostate surgery, we took a trip to the States with my brother, Roger, and his wife, Ruth. (Not only are they fun to be with, Roger loves to do all the driving, and we just go along for the ride!) We wanted to visit some cousins we hadn't seen in a long time, while doing a little cross-border shopping as well.

Before re-entry to Canada, we stopped at Wal-Mart for a few necessities. By "necessities," I'm not referring to the towels Sharon found for our guest bathroom. No, it was actually those men's absorbent pads which I would be needing in just a few weeks and at a cheaper-than-Canadian price.

Throughout my entire life, I had nicely avoided that section of the pharmacy. I'm not sure exactly why, but it probably had to do with the misconception that it was ladies' territory. Television commercials keep us pretty up-to-date on brand names with vague explanation as to their purpose. So I was a bit in the dark. Poise, Depends, Maxi, Equate—who cares?

Interestingly, Roger disappeared after having articulated so precisely what he had found "necessary" and best following his January '08 prostate surgery. I was hoping he would help me in my selection. Instead, he went to fill up on cheaper-than-Canadian gasoline. It apparently hadn't occurred to him to accompany his younger brother on this rather threatening and embarrassing ordeal.

Ruth led the way straight to the pads department, past Depends and over to Equate. She and Sharon seemed so familiar with it all.

"These are for the ladies. Those are for the men."

I'm no dummy. I could at least have figured that out!

"These are for those light days, and these are for the heavy days."

Come on! Is there no mercy?

I couldn't believe this was happening to me. In no time my cart was full and I just wanted to get out of there. But interestingly, Ruth was off looking for other things and Sharon was heading for the towel department. Pushing my well-padded cart, I followed Sharon. I was just glad it didn't have a squeaky wheel. The last thing I needed was to draw attention.

Then Sharon decided a walk would be a good thing since we had spent so much time in the car. The periphery of these huge stores is a good place for a walk; not many people there either. So away we went. I took the lead, pushing my load of men's necessities, with an eye for unwanted crowded areas.

After one round, I realized there was really nowhere to hide. So I proceeded to the checkout area while Sharon did yet another round of exercise. It was only now dawning on me that I had been totally abandoned by my family.

Alone, I went forth muttering to myself, "Too many people there. That line is packed. Why does everyone have to check out exactly when I do?"

Luckily, I found one with no people. Great! The very last thing I wanted was a line of gawkers. You know how everyone stares at the merchandise of everyone else while waiting in line. It's just something to bide the time, I suppose, if not rather entertaining. I wanted no gawkers. But just as I was unloading five big bundles of those babies on the counter, a family appeared out of nowhere—a whole gang of gawkers! I quickly checked out and left, steering toward the exit a hundred yards away.

All alone, I headed to the parking lot, abandoned by everyone dear to me.

From a distance, Roger waved, indicating that he would meet me at the car. From even still farther away, Sharon was gesturing and mouthing that she would find Ruth.

As I wheeled my unseemly load to the car, I noticed that darkness had set in. Yes! Thank God for a cover of darkness. Roger was already there, and I felt a certain bonding with him as I unloaded the cart. Securing everything in the trunk, I began to worry how I might explain my purchases to the customs official.

Finally, with everyone back in the car again, we headed for Canada. Everyone had a good chuckle about my escapade. Roger explained that I will use the larger ones for several weeks after the catheter comes out. Then he went on to tell me I will graduate to the lighter ones, carrying extras in my pocket.

"For how long? Weeks? Months? Years?" I asked.

"It all *Depends*!"

"You guys know it's not Depends I need. Give me a break! I actually bought Equate."

Speaking of Depends, the cycle of life takes us from dependence to independence through interdependence, and all the way back to dependence. The well-promoted manufacturer that created Depends has done us a great favour, as have the other brands, helping us through the later stages of life.

But so did the Psalmist who reminds us that "Those who trust in (depend on) the Lord will lack no good thing" (Psalm 34:10b, NLT). That puts the Lord alongside and above all the "necessities" of life.

Under the Bridge

October 2009

had never been under the bridge before. One day on my favourite river walk along the Thames, I had an urge to check out the grassy trail leading to the bridge. Why? Just curiosity, I guess.

The wet, slippery, uneven path required my full attention as it led downward along the sloping riverbank. As I approached the bridge, I noticed welded wire mesh covering the ground everywhere to prevent erosion. This gave my uncertain footing a new advantage, but I became aware of the constant possibility of tripping on it.

After a few slips and slides, there I was, under the bridge. Why had I come here? This was not an inviting place. Standing there idly, I began to feel chilled in the dampness. My thoughts were scattered and unfocused.

Graffiti covered all the reachable surfaces, even the abutments out in the river. Who put it there? Young people, I presume—perhaps to make a statement or to be remembered. I admired the artistic element of the graffiti but not one word was intelligible to me. Did these colourful gang symbols, or code words, represent rebellion? Perhaps.

Perhaps not. Who am I to judge? I've had my own rebellious moments. I was reminded of a Bible verse—something about God writing my name on something. This is so amazing! God says, "I would not forget you! See, I have written your name on the palms of my hands" (Isaiah 49:15b–16, NLT). I find that rather comforting—God's graffiti!

"Bridge Over Troubled Water" started invading my private thoughts. The water wasn't really troubled, just constantly on the move. It meandered listlessly by with small eddies swirling aimlessly past the large cement abutments, superimposing reflections on the graffiti.

I sensed calmness in my spirit as I stood there alone with my thoughts. No birds twittered. No fish jumped. There weren't even any Canada geese honking or mallard ducks quacking. Silence. Borderline boredom. But those eddies got my attention. They appeared to be trying to fight the current.

"Am I like an eddy?" I wondered. "Resistant? Bucking the reality of the direction of my life? Or are the eddies of my life what keep me from listless, meaningless meandering or, worse yet, stagnation?"

Going back six weeks, my prostate cancer surgery was like an eddy, disrupting the flow of my life. The cancer had extended beyond the prostate, but the surgeon was hopeful that he got everything in the surrounding tissue.

Then, two weeks ago, another eddy landed me in emergency. I came down with a mysterious setback that left me extremely weak and with no appetite while my pain level escalated. I was prescribed an antibiotic for what appeared to be an infection.

One of the four tests they did on me was an ultrasound, which showed a tumour on my kidney. That is eddy number three. Even though today I'm feeling better, tomorrow we meet another specialist to get an idea about what's going on and whether radiation will be needed.

Eddy upon eddy: ongoing resistance to a smooth-flowing life.

I had forgotten, momentarily, that I was under a bridge. It wasn't so silent after all. The continual thump-thudding of traffic overhead, first unnoticed, had become an incessant drone. It was the whirring noise of everyday activity, the constant humming hubbub of people driving places and doing things. Life in the real world was moving forward. There I stood, in my own small world, alone.

Which world do I really prefer? Once again my life is on hold. Or is it? Not really. I'm confident that this is God's plan for my life right now—under the bridge.

During recent years, I've been developing a calm assurance that God is in control of my life. Unlike the bridge, with its erosion-preventing, welded wire mesh, my life has been held together by spiritual supports: the prayer of dear friends and the mercy of our Father in heaven who hears and answers prayer. Whether he answers *yes* or *no* or *wait*, I am in a safe place.

"The LORD is my rock, my fortress, and my savior; my God is my rock, in whom I find protection. He is my shield, the power that saves me, and my place of safety" (Psalm 18:2, NLT).

Under-the-bridge perspective has helped me refocus on who I am, where I am, and God's care for me. I doubt I will ever visit there again. I've seen enough to whet my curiosity.

Shortly after sending this story out to my contact list, one of our dear friends sent me this note of encouragement:

When I received your story Under the Bridge, I wrote a little poem expressing what I heard in your story. So, I am taking the liberty of forwarding it to you. Hope you find it interesting.

Blessings,
Glenn Taylor (4 Mary 2)

UNDER THE BRIDGE

Attracted by curiosity (or God) to a new place
Unstable, slippery ground, secured by mesh.
Graffiti spoken to deaf, unresponsive concrete,
Perhaps, because not heard by ears of flesh.

God was there, my name upon His palms.
Those loving hands bring swirls into my life,
Eddies of meaning, purpose, intention, disruption,
Yet, meaningful for He is present in the strife.

The world does not stop, unaware of me,
Thumping-thudding, whirring through each day.
Sometimes great distance separates the hubbub,
But, God shields and protects, is with us in the fray.

Glenn Taylor, October 2009
Used by permission.

Good News, Bad News

December 2009

G ood news, bad news. You win, you lose.
One of these scenarios paid me a visit last week.
(Or should that be *scenarii*, for some of you etymologists?) On November 28, the same symptoms I had in mid-October returned: no appetite, no energy, chills and sweats, an annoying cough, and increased muscle pain. I just plain felt sick! And to frustrate the doctors, I had no temperature.

Back in October, we ended up going to our local hospital emergency. Seven hours later, they asked us to return the next day for an ultrasound, assuming there was a post-op infection from my prostatectomy in September.

Next day, four hours later, we were sent home with an antibiotic that seemed to do the trick. That was good. I started my walking routine again. Some energy returned, and I even did a live presentation of *Choose Joy: Philippians in Person*. Getting more or less back on track felt really good.

Then boom! The same symptoms returned. This time the urology department moved up an already scheduled CT scan and x-ray to December 2. Two days later, they told us that my condition had nothing to do with urology. Good news! That's great. I could relax knowing there were no complications from the surgery. But it didn't change the fact that I still felt lousy.

Our family doctor saw me as soon as an appointment could be arranged. After taking my temperature, he said, "No temperature. But I believe you have the flu."

"We've already had the H1N1 flu shot," I clarified.

He went on to explain, "This particular flu lasts for weeks, and then takes weeks for a full recovery. You probably had it before you got the shot."

Bad news! We had to cancel a number of family and seasonal events as well as some scheduled *OASIS* programs.

I did some web browsing and discovered that it's possible to have H1N1 with no temperature. I don't know if that was good news or bad news for me. In any case I was feeling a bit better, and that was good news!

I always try to keep my stories somewhat upbeat and encouraging. So far, this one is downright depressing! Sorry. But here's the scoop. We all face good news–bad news scenarios. They may relate to health or finances or relationships; sometimes they require immediate action. Other times they leave one facing a dilemma.

Don't you hate it when someone says, "Which do you want first, the good news or the bad news?" Either way, you win, you lose. Or do you?

The book of Philippians has impacted me so deeply. Having memorized it and presented it often in public, I am always challenged and blessed. God actually speaks to me through it every time.

Today, I can't escape the apostle Paul's statement in Philippians 4:12, "I have learned to be content, whatever the circumstances. I know what it is to be in need. And I know what it is to have plenty. I have learned the secret of being content in any and every situation."

I know what it is to be sick. And I know what it is to be well. But I'm still working on the *contentment* part. The secret? He tells us in verse 13: "I can do all this through Him, who gives me strength."

That's it! That's exactly what I needed. Thank you for wandering through this anecdote with me. Jesus will strengthen and help me as I trust Him. He will do the same for you too.

Lessons in Snow

February 2010

Forgive me, but I love snow. Fifty years ago tobogganing on the hills of our farm was a favourite winter pastime. The closest I came to skiing and snowboarding was tobogganing standing up. It's a wonder I didn't break my neck!

These days, however, occasionally shovelling off our driveway is about my only encounter with snow. I do enjoy the exercise, even though one of the perks of condo living is having all that done for us.

My preference is looking at snow out the window. As I sit here in our front room, the sunlight is glistening on the drifts across the roadway. Beautiful! The brighter the sun, the bluer the shadows! Have you ever noticed that? Shadows in the snow are often a bluish colour.

Supposing snow represented our lives? Would it be white or blue? Sunny or shadowy? I reckon God gives both to keep us balanced.

What really gets my attention is the exquisite beauty of a solitary snowflake. More beautiful than the snowscape of an open field or billowing drifts along the highway, a single snowflake has character and form that is unparalleled.

Yesterday as I sat in my car while Sharon did some shopping, I was enamoured by big fluffy flakes of snow gently landing on the window beside me. I turned to watch them glide to a stop, rest awhile, then quickly melt away because of the warmth of the window. I took a closer look, singling out individual snowflakes, watching them glisten in the sunlight. Then from the tiny tips inward, they gradually turned to water. What a shame. Oh, how I wanted them to stay longer. There was so much detail to be examined—each flake different, yet similar, with six points extending outward from the complex center. No artist in the world could ever reproduce the splendour of this delicate crystal lattice, so intricately woven together.

Then poof! Only a drop of water remained.

There are many lessons in snow. Snow means different things to different people: To the ski industry, snow means success. To the skier, it means fun. To the city council, it means expenditure. For snow removal crews, it's income. To an artist, snow means inspiration. To those who live on the edge of a mountain, danger.

Yet nature looks to snow for help. To ground vegetation, snow is a warm blanket. To a glacier, snow means growth as it piles up, presses down and turns into ice.

Oh yes, one more lesson: "Though your sins are like scarlet, they shall be as white as snow" (Isaiah1:18). God says so. His forgiveness is so immense!

Where does snow come from? We know the weather brings it on. Scientific things happen in the skies, and it snows. But God asked Job this question: "Have you entered the storehouses of the snow?" (Job 38:22).

My answer: "Never—except for those little snow forts we made when we were kids, where we stored our stash of snowballs."

According to Psalm 147:16 (NLT), "God sends the snow like white wool; he scatters frost upon the ground like ashes." Thank you, God. Your creation is awesome.

Where do the snowflakes go? They land. They melt. They vaporize. In one sense, they live forever in those three states. In the big scheme of things, our life, like a snowflake on the window, is the same.

In James 4:14 we read, "What is your life? You are a mist that appears for a little while and then vanishes." We are born. We live. We die. But our soul lives on forever. Eternity is part of God's plan for us.

One day back in my tobogganing years, I asked Jesus to forgive my sin and be my Saviour and Lord. I wanted to be sure that I would go to heaven when I die. Today I live with gratitude for the gift of God, "Eternal life in Jesus Christ our Lord" (Romans 6:23b).

You know what? Whether our life is grand and glistening white in the glory of good times, or whether we're in the dull and blue shadows of challenge and discouragement, we are beautiful to God. He loves us way more than I love the snow. And that's a lot!

"Keep yourselves in God's love as you wait for the mercy of our Lord Jesus Christ to bring you to eternal life" (Jude 1:21).

White Winter Sonnet

White Winter wind beguiles the Autumn hue,
And whistles wildly o'er the frozen fields.
While wearily waiting Spring and Summer dew,
The brittle, icy grass its lustre yields.

Faint chirps the chickadee from nestled hutch,
While cocky jay and cardinal steal their fare.
Surviving blizzard, shivering homeless crouch,
Refusing shelter from the frigid air.

White Winter 'waits the adolescent Spring.
Nor can the youthful Summer rid its blow,
As ageing Fall anticipates the sting
Of death, of cold, of frost and blinding snow.

Why worry we of Winter, white and cold?
For Christ our Saviour loves us, young or old.

© 2008, David Gast

33—66—99

March 2010

What I'm about to say has nothing to do with web-safe colours, though I was intrigued to discover that 33, 66, and 99 are part of a compatible colour code for website construction.

Thirty-three is an intriguing and somewhat popular number. In my case, it was the number of radiation treatments I required for prostate cancer, decided upon by my radiologist. I was pretty sure it didn't have anything to do with my age, even though I was thirty-three in sixty-six because I was born in forty-four! I will be sixty-six this year! Maybe they decided that the number of half my age was all the radiation I should have!

Seriously speaking, thirty-three seemed to be a very common number among many of the patients I talked to in the waiting room. One man said that those who had undergone prostate surgery typically got thirty-three. Several others, however, were receiving thirty-five or more. A friend of mine in Toronto needed forty.

So I Googled it and found out that the dose of radiation therapy is the key factor, not the number of treatments. The area being treated is prescribed a "total dose" of radiation—usually close to the lifetime maximum that that area of the body can tolerate. Because radiation would be very toxic if given in one big dose, it is divided (fractionated) into smaller, better-tolerated doses. In my case, I needed thirty-three.

So now we know. Thirty-three is not a magical number. It is simply the fractionated dose. And it works. Those who are experts in this field say that low doses of radiation over a period of time damage the DNA of cancerous cells. Normal cells are able to quickly repair this damage before dividing, but cancerous cells cannot. Since prostate cancer grows slowly, many weeks of therapy are necessary to continually damage the cancerous cells, preventing them from repairing themselves.

I know it works because I've been there. I was eleven in fifty-five! I had thyroid cancer—very serious and very rare for a child. After surgery, they radiated my entire neck area with "the cobalt bomb." That's what they called it!

I was intrigued this past January when I walked into the waiting area of the London Health Sciences Centre. There, in the middle of the room, was a mural of the history of radiation in London, Ontario, and a picture of the machine that treated me in 1955. I feel like I'm part of the history—a survivor. Radiation does work.

Yes, it's true. So far I've survived thyroid cancer, lung cancer, skin cancer and prostate cancer. I told someone recently that it seems like I'm trying them all out!

As of today I feel great with only one of the thirty-three radiation treatments remaining. Side effects have been minimal. I feel better now than I did when the treatments started. I have so much to be thankful for.

And I'm thankful to the Lord for His ongoing presence and help through my cancer journeys. He promises to be with us and never forsake us. That's confirmed by the Psalmist, David. "Even when I walk through the darkest valley, I will not be afraid, for you are close beside me" (Psalm 23:4, NLT).

God sent His Son, Jesus Christ, to live in our world for thirty-three years. He spent thirty-three years showing us what God looks like, teaching us truth, and demonstrating His divine love and grace. At the end of administering that Dose of Divine Therapy, Jesus died for our sin and rose from the dead for our salvation. Now He lives in the hearts of all who believe in Him.

Imagine this. In thirty-three years, 2043, I will either be ninety-nine, or I'll be home in heaven with Jesus. How good is that?

Unwelcome Visitors

April 2010

April—One of my favourite months! The weather has been superb. Spring sprang unseasonably warm and early this year, sending winter on a fast retreat, leaving buds and blossoms bursting before their time. How beautiful! How exhilarating and encouraging!

The warm weather and spring flowers are welcome visitors. They make me want to be out in the garden, working. But my inner voice keeps whispering, "Don't be in a hurry. It's not even May yet. One has to build up one's energy after such a difficult fall and winter!"

However, since my prostate surgery in September, my life has been totally disrupted by unwelcome visitors. You know—the kind that arrive and wear out their welcome very quickly, leaving you wishing they would just go away! They have drained my energy and tried my patience.

No, they weren't family or friends. Our family and friends can come and stay as long as they like, any time. Matter of fact, Marty and Holly, our cruise-ship-entertainer son and daughter-in-law spent a week with us here in London, and last month we spent a week with them in their new condo in the States. What a great time we had!

Except for unwelcome visitor number five. That's right. I said, *five*! You see, there had been six of these characters altogether—one a month: two bouts of the flu in October and November, two colds in January and February, and two more really nasty colds in March and April. Cough, cough. Sniff, sniff. Blow, blow.

The thirty-three radiation treatments I received, from January 27 to March 16, were nothing compared to these ugly, unwanted intruders. Three times since October, antibiotics were prescribed with the intention of sending my nasty maladies packing, but to no avail.

Sharon and I were both hoping to be in good voice for our *OASIS* singing group, with eight gigs on the books before the end of May. On top of that, four dramatic monologue presentations of *Choose Joy: Philippians in Person* were scheduled for the same time frame.

Sharon got through our first program, having had laryngitis only days before. We are presently in the midst of these events and gradually our voices are clearing up. It seems that God is giving us just enough voice to sing in each presentation, and people are kindly expressing appreciation for the blessing received.

Singing in *OASIS* with Frank and Brenda has been a refreshing part of our life during these months. An oasis is actually an area of fertile ground in a desert where the underground water has risen to ground level and where plants grow and travelers can replenish water supplies. Getting together to sing and prepare our programs is an oasis for each of us. We hope it's the same for the many seniors groups where we present our program.

An oasis is also a place, or period of time, that gives relief from a troubling or chaotic situation. Our recent wilderness of colds and flu has been our chaotic situation—our desert. We have had to ask God, over and over, to replenish our capacity to sing.

Jesus said, "Come to me all you who are weary and carry heavy burdens, and I will give you rest" (Matthew 11:28,

NLT). As we turn to the Lord Jesus, the True Oasis, He refreshes our spirit, soul, and body.

Now, about that untended garden? I'll get to it someday. Once this last intruder is gone, and I've coughed my last cough, I'll be ready and willing to get my hands dirty and spruce up our tiny condo gardens with cheery flowers and plants—definitely welcome visitors to our premises.

His Spring
Sonnet

Forgotten are the dull, dark, dreary days.
Pure joy of spring time floods the azure sky.
At rising sun through glorious, golden rays
Song sparrows, flitting, sing and fly.

Once hidden, now revealed for all to see,
The barren branches, bent from frigid strife,
Now breathe, through bursting buds, new energy.
With winter finally gone, life comes to life.

Rejoice, O resurrected, emerald earth.
Be glad and sing, O weary one. Revive!
It is a gift, this treasure of new birth,
For me, forevermore alive!

From death to death cold winter came and went.
From death to life His spring our LORD has sent.

© 2011, David Gast

Bearers of Good News

May 2010

We sometimes say, "No news is good news." Maybe that's true, but it leaves you at the mercy of information you don't have. And what you don't know often becomes a springboard for assumption.

A communications teacher once told me never to assume anything. He said, "To 'assume' makes an 'ass' out of 'u' and 'me'!" That's a little crass, but he was probably justified in giving this advice. To base assertions on partial information is simply guessing, and guessing can lead us down the wrong path very quickly.

Last week, I had my regular six-month consultation with the oncologist relating to my lung cancer. I always go to these sessions with some trepidation. This was five years after chemotherapy. I remember my surgeon telling us at the onset of my lung cancer journey in 2004, that with chemotherapy following surgery, my chance of survival could increase significantly after five years. That seemed like good news, not based on assumption, but rather on the results of many case studies.

First thing, upon arriving at the clinic, I was sent for a blood test. That was followed by a chest x-ray. During these procedures and the waiting time before the doctor arrived, I was quietly praying that God would grant me good news. But being somewhat weak in faith, I braced myself for the worst and hoped for the best.

Finally I was led to the consultation room, interviewed by a nurse and left there alone, waiting and wondering which doctor it would be—Dr. Y. or his assistant, Dr. N.

An attractive female Asian doctor, whom I had never met before, suddenly entered and introduced herself as Dr. L., Dr. Y.'s intern. She sat down, opened my chart, and in an enthusiastic tone of voice said, "I have good news for you. You are cured. There is no evidence of your cancer recurring, so we will not need to see you again."

She's got to be kidding, I thought to myself. My head was spinning. *How is it that an intern I don't know can be the bearer of this incredible news? Do I believe her or not? Is she experienced enough? Does she really know my case well enough to make this diagnosis?*

I tried to articulate the only question that sprang to mind. "Would it be good for me to get a second opinion from my original surgeon and oncologist in Orillia?"

Attempting to put me at ease, she softly asked, "Why would you want a second opinion? The x-ray is clear. Questionable spots on the x-ray that have been tracked for five years have not changed. And protocol is that after two years they are considered noncancerous."

She paused, then continued. "But it is not uncommon for people who are cured to go through a time of disbelief with a feeling of being suddenly lost, wondering, 'Who is going to look after me now?'"

I was still processing her reassurance after she left the room to get Dr. Y. Time seemed to stand still.

Together, they returned. Dr. Y. reached out and shook my hand, a broad smile on his face. "You are a very lucky man. I have only said this to a handful of lung cancer patients in my whole career. *Your lung cancer is cured.*"

This is actually the second time I have heard that my cancer was cured. The first was in 1966, ten years after my thyroid cancer. I thank God for his healing grace—again. I am indebted to the many people who prayed for me. And I am grateful to the team of medical people including researchers, technicians, doctors, nurses, support staff, and who-knows-who-else behind the scenes. With two cancers down, now we concentrate on the other two: prostate and skin. To "assume" anything about them would—well, let's not go there!

Good news is always way better than no news.

I'm glad I heard and believed the good news of salvation when I was a young boy. Jesus calls it the gospel, and I still believe it. In Romans 1:16, we read that it *is the power of God that brings salvation to everyone who believes.*

Our future in heaven is secured through believing the good news that God loves us. Here is a thought from Romans 10: "How beautiful are the feet of bearers of good news!"

That is so true. But in a similar way the same goes for Dr. L. and Dr. Y.

Invested Grace

August 2010

Ve all know life has its challenges. It is part of being human. One day my research on the Internet revealed an article by Rachelle Disbennett Lee titled *Obstacles Can Be Opportunities in Disguise.* I suppose that's correct. She said that *obstacles are the U-turns in life that help us find a new path.* That statement got me thinking.

As obstacles come, we have a choice: we can either go through them alone or with God's help turn them into opportunities.

Here's how it works. A tough obstacle arrives. We say, "God help me!"

God says, "My grace is sufficient for you, for my power is made perfect in weakness" (2 Corinthians 12:9). He doesn't always take our problems away. He invests His grace in us to help us go through the tough stuff. We are encouraged. We go on living life, viewing our situation as an opportunity to give glory to God and to encourage others.

Over the years, I have shared a lot about my health journey—maybe too much to the point of boredom. May I impinge on your patience once more as we focus on the grace of God? As a boy, in 1955, I underwent surgery for thyroid cancer, followed by cobalt radiation. After ten years of checkups, I was pronounced cured. In late 2004, lung cancer was discovered. The lower lobe of my right lung was surgically removed, followed by chemotherapy. After five years of surveillance, I was declared clear of lung cancer. Praise God!

My being healed of cancer twice is a God-thing—a gift of undeserved grace. It had nothing to do with who I am or what I have done. God is investing grace in me by *carrying on to completion the work He began in me.* See Philippians 1:6. So here I am, alive and well, by His grace.

I still have two cancers being watched and treated as well as a spot on my kidney. Two skin cancers were dealt with surgically last week. Another was removed with liquid nitrogen. Prostate cancer, discovered in 2009, led to surgery and radiation treatments. Though a surveillance schedule is set up for the next number of years, a recent checkup indicated a PSA of zero. You can't get much better than that! Another experience of God's invested grace in me.

Today I'm wondering why. Why should I receive what I do not deserve? What should my response be?

For starters, my response is one of giving glory to God. These cancers could have taken my life, but for some reason, God in His sovereign grace has chosen to protect and heal me. He has chosen to answer, in the affirmative, the prayers of many friends and family. My heart overflows with thanksgiving to God. I thank Him for extending my life, for His presence with me on the journey, and for the certainty that someday He will complete the work He has begun in me by taking me home to heaven.

Another response is that of giving back to God, though it's not required of us to do so. God has no strings attached to His investments. God's invested grace is a gift undeserved, unearned, irrevocable, and not based on returns. But it has been a privilege for Sharon and me to make returns on God's investment in our lives by sharing our cancer journey with others. Through our singing and sharing, we have been able to invest grace in the lives of others, bringing encouragement and seeking to inspire a deeper sense of hope and faith in God.

I realize that I have been the recipient of God's invested grace. His grace has been more than enough to carry me through the unknowns and uncertainties. I'm beginning to see the bigger picture, gaining fresh *perspective*. Sometimes God heals us. Sometimes He doesn't. If I go on living indefinitely, that's good. If I don't, that's even better because His saving grace will take me to a much better place.

Grace for living. Grace for dying. His grace is sufficient.

The choice is ours. Receive the investment or go it alone. Yes, we can all choose to experience the grace of the Lord Jesus Christ—both His saving grace as well as the grace He gives for facing life's daily challenges. Simply by asking, it will be given, and those obstacles will become opportunities.

Deep Summer Heat
Sonnet

Deep summer heat 'neath shimmering molten sky;
Suspended dust tornados whirl and run.
Brown shriveled grasses wither, brittle dry,
Dehydrated by blast of deadly sun.

When heat is on, not from the sun in space,
But rather, heat of conflict, loss, or pain,
Far deadlier is the consequence we face.
For not just he who struggles is to blame.

All hope seems stifled without solace, shade.
Who can such torrid tribulation stand?
Who can endure this life, yet unafraid
Move on to face each day in its demand?

Sweet summer shade, cool waters bathe the soul
Of those who make the love of God their goal.

Shadow-Talk

September 2010

Morning walks are the best. Cool. Exhilarating. What a way to start a day! One morning, while heading west on Killaly, I became aware of my shadow. I've seen my shadow umpteen times. This time, the fact that my shadow was ahead of me got me thinking.

The thing that interested me was the fact that my shadow never left me. It shifted position, however, depending on what direction I took. It preceded me whenever I was walking away from the sun and followed me when I walked toward the sun. Going west or east, whatever my direction, there it was.

"Go west, old man. Follow your shadow. But don't trip on it!" What a bizarre notion! Here I am, following my shadow. Does that put me somehow in the past in relation to my shadow?

"Shadow of the past." Somewhere, at some forgotten time in my life, I've heard those words. So what's this all about? Do they have a deeper meaning? Do shadows somehow symbolize my past—or part of it?

No. Let's not get philosophical. Shadows plainly mean I'm going west!

Let me get this straight. I'm neither moving forward to the past nor would I be heading back to the future if I turned around. I am in the moment, moving west along Killaly, enjoying a morning walk. Simple as that. And that is exactly how I view my life—in the moment. "Now" is of far greater importance than anything ahead of or behind me.

Intrigued, I pondered, "What exactly is a shadow?"

Shadows merely indicate that light is present. Wikipedia says a shadow is an area where direct light cannot shine due to obstruction by an object.

Okay, I get it. I'm the barrier! I am the obstruction standing in the way of the light.

Oh no! That sounds awful! I didn't go for a walk to get depressed. But when you think about it, that puts shadows in a whole new light. Sorry for the pun!

Then I thought about the dark side. There *is* a dark side, you know. Shadows have often been synonymous with the foreboding side of life. Alfred Hitchcock used shadows skillfully to portray suspense and intrigue.

Did you know there are people who are spooked by their own shadow? They suffer from *sciophobia* or *sciaphobia* if your shadow is a female. And a person who is "living in someone else's shadow" is somewhat diminished in significance and influence.

Shadows aren't always a negative thing, however. They can be a refreshing place on a hot and humid day. In a sentimental 1905 song, a jilted lover consoles himself, *"In the shade of the old apple tree."* That's cool!

Shadows are also useful. Although they were instrumental in telling time back when sun dials were in vogue, I have no ability in telling time from shadows. There have been occasions, however, when I have used shadows to help me figure out in what direction I was going. In that regard, shadows are very helpful.

In 1 John, a short book near the end of the Bible, we are encouraged to *"walk in the light."* This is not referring to the sun, but to God. "God is light; in Him there is no darkness at all" (1 John 1:5). His light does not produce shadows but is absorbed in those who are in the Light, and who then reflect that Light to others.

Jesus said, "I have come into the world as a light, so that no one who believes in me should stay in darkness" (John 12:46). Only by obstructing the light through disbelief are we left in dark shadows.

Following a competent worker in on-the-job training is called shadowing. In the same way, I want to be found shadowing Jesus who said, "I am the light of the world. Whoever follows me will never walk in darkness, but will have the light of life" (John 8:12). What a wonderful promise for His shadowers!

Killaly, maybe I'll be back tomorrow. Enough shadow-talk for today.

Here's something to think about. "Whatever is good and perfect comes down to us from God our Father, who created all the lights in the heavens. He never changes or casts a shifting shadow" (James 1:17, NLT).

Keeping Track

January 2011

I get great joy from making lists and keeping track of all kinds of things. For me, creating spreadsheets on the computer is great fun. Really! Lists help me organize my life. They indicate changes and trends. What would life have been like if I had pursued a career involving data entry or accounting? Accounting would not have worked. Definitely not! Ask Sharon, who is our self-appointed family budget guardian! But data entry may have been a possibility.

One example is my document that tracks all our car expenses: fuel, maintenance, insurance. It also shows the cost per kilometre averaged over the life of our 2003 Toyota. Up to this point, the car has cost us twenty-two cents per kilometre. According to my calculations, gas averaged $.97 per litre in 2010. This year we are already at $1.12, indicating that what seemed painful last year isn't nearly as painful as it will be this year. That's really important information, don't you think?

Here's another example. Since retiring, and actually for several years before, I have kept track of medical appointments and procedures. The last three years show an interesting trend: 2008, twelve; 2009, forty-eight; 2010, ninety-one. Yikes! Of course thirty-three of the ninety-one were radiation treatments.

Did you know that God is a list maker too? He writes the names of His followers in His Book of Life. "Rejoice that your names are written in heaven" (Luke 10:20, NIV).

Discover anew, in Psalm 139, God's detailed knowledge of us. In it He says that He has even written down exactly how many days we will live from the moment of conception. And imagine this: "The very hairs of your head are all numbered" (Luke 12:7).

According to suffering Job, God even counts our steps. "Surely then, you will count my steps but not keep track of my sin" (Job 14:16, NIV).

I heard last week that we should be taking ten thousand steps a day in order to keep healthy. I'll leave the step counting up to God! I don't have a pedometer, but I do keep a spreadsheet for my walking with date, minutes, and distance covered, calculating the average speed. Interestingly, for some reason, a slowing trend has evolved. As a matter of fact, I realized the other day that I have not had that document open for a couple of months due to an acute back problem, going way beyond the sciatica that I have endured for a dozen years. I'll be keeping my physiotherapist busy for quite a while.

My most recent list helps me monitor pain medication. This is of paramount importance because of my poor memory. To keep from overdosing, I designed a chart where I record the date, time, and medication taken.

Thank God that He knows all about me. "You keep track of all my sorrows. You have collected all my tears in your bottle. You have recorded each one in your book" (Psalm 56:8, NLT).

Whatever is of utmost importance to Him, He writes down—certainly not because of a poor memory, but because He loves me. It brings me comfort to know He keeps track of me.

PSALM 139

O LORD, you have examined my heart and know everything about me. You know when I sit down or stand up. You know my thoughts even when I'm far away. You see me when I travel and when I rest at home. You know everything I do. You know what I am going to say even before I say it, LORD. You go before me and follow me. You place your hand of blessing on my head. Such knowledge is too wonderful for me, too great for me to understand!

I can never escape from your Spirit! I can never get away from your presence! If I go up to heaven, you are there; if I go down to the grave, you are there. If I ride the wings of the morning, if I dwell by the farthest oceans, even there your hand will guide me, and your strength will support me. I could ask the darkness to hide me and the light around me to become night—but even in darkness I cannot hide from you. To you the night shines as bright as day. Darkness and light are the same to you.

You made all the delicate, inner parts of my body and knit me together in my mother's womb. Thank you for making me so wonderfully complex! Your workmanship is marvelous—how well I know it. You watched me as I was being formed in utter seclusion, as I was woven together in the dark of the womb. You saw me before I was born. Every day of my life was recorded in your book. Every moment was laid out before a single day had passed.

How precious are your thoughts about me, O God. They cannot be numbered! I can't even count them; they outnumber the grains of sand! And when I wake up, you are still with me!

O God, if only you would destroy the wicked! Get out of my life, you murderers! They blaspheme you; your enemies misuse your name. O LORD, shouldn't I hate those who hate you? Shouldn't I despise those who oppose you? Yes, I hate them with total hatred, for your enemies are my enemies.

Search me, O God, and know my heart; test me and know my anxious thoughts. Point out anything in me that offends you, and lead me along the path of everlasting.

Psalm 139, NLT

The Cheese Challenge

April 4, 2011

Cheese is a favourite food of mine. Cheddar, gouda, feta and even cottage cheese—it's all good. I love it. Yesterday I picked up a book I had read back in 2000 called *Who Moved My Cheese?* (by Spencer Johnson, 1998). It's a good read—an allegory of how to deal with change in your life. Two mice, Sniff and Scurry, and two tiny people, Hem and Haw, go searching for cheese in a maze and find a great stash. But one day the cheese mysteriously disappears. While in search of new cheese, the natural instincts of the mice prove far superior to the mental and emotional tactics of the tiny people. The cheese represents what is really important in our life—what makes us feel successful and fulfilled.

That book was required reading in one of my new ministry assignments a number of years ago. For me, my "cheese" was my job. That is what gave me self-worth. What I did was synonymous with who I was. If I were to tell you about my life, it would be a list of all the jobs and ministries I have had.

Then everything changed. Somebody moved my cheese! Health challenges brought my church music ministry to a screeching halt. Lung cancer, prostate cancer, skin cancer, an ongoing severe back pain, and now recent concern over a tumour on one of my kidneys, have all demanded a lot of time and attention. I sometimes worry whether my health has become "my cheese"—my identity. People seem more interested in how I am rather than what I have done. Conversations are often organ recitals, both mine and theirs!

Like Hem and Haw, I have longed for the old cheese. I've hemmed and hawed about what to do with the rest of my life, sometimes wishing I could go back a few years!

Sniff and Scurry adapted to change quickly. They took off immediately to find new cheese. The book says that the quicker you let go of old cheese, the sooner you can enjoy new cheese. Actually, I have been a bit like Sniff. After sniffing out some job possibilities, I discarded them all because my medical schedule and condition would have interfered.

Then I realized I already had three significant "cheeses" on the go. Opportunities still arise for me to present *Choose Joy: Philippians in Person*. Also, our group *OASIS* is facing a busy schedule. The third opportunity is volunteering as a conversational English facilitator with immigrant people. These all energize and motivate me.

The cheese scouts were also given this word of advice: "Savour the adventure and the taste of the new cheese." And I do, I really do!

There is much more for me to savour. Psalm 34:8 says, "Oh taste and see that the Lord is good."

Recently, I rediscovered a new chunk of cheese in the marvelous maze of scripture. It's the one I remember my father quoting many times.

"Those who hope in the Lord will renew their strength. They will soar on wings like eagles; they will run and not grow weary, they will walk and not be faint" (Isaiah 40:31).

Now that's who I want to be—a person energized by faith in God. Whenever I hope and trust in God, my stability isn't shaken by every new medical test or doctor's consultation. He renews my inner strength. I can soar. I can run. I can walk.

What is really important to me now? What is my true identity? Certainly not my job. I don't have one! Not my health. It's not very dependable. My identity is found in my relationship with Jesus Christ. I am His and He is mine. He is the strength of my life. He is my song. He has become my salvation. In Him I find forgiveness, peace, and joy. As I put my hope and trust in Him, He dishes out life abundant, real life, eternal life, meaningful and fulfilled life.

Thank you, I'll take that. Yes, Lord, maybe with a dash of fresh parmesan!

Diminishing Returns

August 2011

They say 85 percent of people have had a bad back at least once in their lifetime. So chances are, you're one of them. For several decades I have visited physiotherapists and chiropractors, receiving a ton of help. Just about the time I think I'm fit and fine, I overdo something and back I go again. You'd think I'd learn!

Last November I picked up something incorrectly. Having grown up on a farm, I know the right and wrong way to lift heavy objects. But this time I acted impulsively and reached to lift while stooping over. I knew better, but Mr. Macho Muscleman thought he could handle it! Too much was too much. The law of diminishing returns kicked in and the result was major pain, loss of mobility, and the need to avoid lifting anything heavier than my shoes.

After months of therapy, my physiotherapist told me that my back was the best she had seen it in over two years. Progress was obvious. So, thinking it would be okay to lift a bit more, I helped Sharon with the groceries, which included a case of water bottles. Woops!

Unfortunately, the fire of our hope often gets rained on by the law of diminishing returns, the origin of which is in economics. The law of diminishing returns forecasts an actual decline in profits when too much positive input is injected into a project. For example, where the addition of one extra person on an assembly line may increase production, three may put it in the red. In other words, it's possible to have too much of a good thing. Moderate lifting helps strengthen our muscles. A case of water bottles sent me back for more therapy.

There's a tipping point where the law of diminishing returns kicks in. It could be somewhere between nibbling on a few potato chips and wolfing down a whole bag. Soaking in the rays for half an hour on the beach can be therapeutic whereas three hours may result in a nasty sunburn. Fertilizer improves crop production, but too much will reduce the yield. Something I have been dealing with is trying to discover the point at which it no longer makes sense to keep fixing an old car. In so many areas of life it is important to figure out the tipping point.

Consider food. I'm bothered in restaurants where portions are so huge that most people can't finish what is served, while famine is ravaging the lives of tens of thousands in the horn of Africa. I am also bothered by my own lack of discretion and control at all-you-can-eat buffets. When is too much too much? There is a tipping point in every meal where one more mouthful is counterproductive. From that point on there are diminishing returns: weight gain, health problems, waste.

You've heard the expression "less is more." When I step on the scale, I often wish that more was less! I'd like to see some diminishing returns there where the numbers are diminishing and my weight is returning to what it was in high school.

Recently, we were commenting on the fact that we consume far too much sugar, too much fat, way too much salt, and too much food in general! In moderation, pretty much anything can be okay; too much of most things isn't.

Or is it? I've been thinking about that. Are there areas of life where too much does not exist? Think about this.

Virtue cannot be overdone. Love, joy, peace, patience, kindness, goodness, faithfulness, gentleness, and self-control are all doable and good and cannot be overdone. They build character into our lives and strength into our relationships. There are no diminishing returns in any of them.

Prayer is another one. Whoever heard of excessive prayer? There are no diminishing returns with prayer. Look at these tremendous words from Jesus:

> Keep on asking, and you will receive what you ask for. Keep on seeking, and you will find. Keep on knocking, and the door will be opened to you. For everyone who asks, receives. Everyone who seeks, finds. And to everyone who knocks, the door will be opened. You parents—if your children ask for a loaf of bread, do you give them a stone instead? Or if they ask for a fish, do you give them a snake? Of course not! So if you sinful people know how to give good gifts to your children, how much more will your heavenly Father give good gifts to those who ask him.
>
> Matthew 7:7–11 (NLT)

What about God's grace? Grace is what God does for us that we don't deserve and cannot earn. Salvation is a gift of God's grace. "For it is by grace you have been saved, through faith—and this is not from yourselves, it is the gift of God—not by works, so that no one can boast" (Ephesians 2:8–9). Is there some fixed limit on what God has done, or will do, for those who believe that Jesus died for our sin and rose again, offering abundant and eternal life?

Gradually, I'm getting my head around it all. But there's a point where too much thinking gets me confused. There it is again—diminishing returns in action! One thing that I'm not confused about is Mr. Macho Muscleman. That's who I need *not* be. Nor is it who I am or ever will be.

THE WEB
SONNET

Intimidating master of the loom
Weaves silent symmetry in silken thread
A web, unseen, in sullen heat of noon.
What morsel unaware will meet its dread?

How delicate the diamond dewdrops shine.
As glistening grid of silver coated lace
Displays the handiwork of the Divine,
In concert with the wonder of His grace.

What web wove we through our productive years?
What legacy of blessing, or of pain?
Soft safety net dispelling hurt and fears?
Or trap of loss, resentment and disdain?

Serve God and man with grace and dignity.
Your web is your responsibility.

© 2008, David Gast

Living with Limitations

November 2011

Handling limitations is tough and goes against my nature. I want to be involved in life. Make exciting plans. Be able and free to travel. Choose activities that bring meaning and purpose. But boundaries, due to my health history, hem me in. For me, being at ease in my shrinking world is a challenge.

It behooves me to take seriously the words I so often quote from Philippians, chapter 4, about learning *"to be content in any and every situation."* That's obviously good advice, a noble and worthwhile lesson. But putting feet on it is another matter. I am too much inclined to resist limitations and complain. Whenever that happens, life isn't pretty and I'm not much fun to be around!

Another opportunity came up for me to present *Choose Joy: Philippians in Person*, but it was back to back with one of our *OASIS* Christmas concerts. My loving wife, Sharon, knows me all too well and insisted I turn down the invitation. It was so hard for me to accept the wisdom of her tough love and even more difficult to have to decline the invitation.

My head said, "No problem. Go for it!"

My body whimpered, "Yes, let's give it a try."

Wisdom asserted, "Don't push it. Accept your limitations and be content."

I'd like to say that I automatically "chose joy" and accepted the reality of my limited energy. But the whole matter weighed heavily upon me and self-pity began to surface.

There are practical ways to pull out of the doldrums. Let a day or two go by. Pray for a renewed spirit of hope. Gain perspective on the bigger picture. In Lord of the Rings, Tolkien said, *"From the ashes a fire shall be woken, a light from the shadows shall spring."* Could it be so?

As our plans were discussed and adjusted, the *Choose Joy* presentation was rescheduled, my limitations were lifted, and so were my spirits!

Speaking of limitations, I share briefly in our regular *OASIS* program about my cancer journey, which now totals five different and unrelated cancers. Most recently, kidney cancer has been added to the list. Treatment begins in mid-December, and through renal radiofrequency ablation the doctors are very optimistic the tumours will be successfully eliminated. As for the other cancers, they are no longer a present threat, for which I give grateful praise to God and thanksgiving to our excellent medical resources and personnel.

Here are three lessons this slow learner has been trying to get a grip on. Some are quotes from my book, *Musing and Muttering through Cancer*. But the Bible is my best and most reliable resource for life and for living with limitations:

1. Today is a special gift from God. The key thing that I'm still trying to learn is to glean God's best for me each day by accepting His schedule and His events in His good time. "Teach us to number our days, that we may gain a heart of wisdom. Satisfy us in the morning with your unfailing love, that we may sing for joy and be glad all our days" (Psalm 90:12, 14).

2. God loves me even when I'm ticked off. *"Ticked Off"* is the title of a chapter in *Musing and Muttering through Cancer*. On one of my very worst days during chemotherapy, back in 2005, I discovered a very encouraging verse. It's like a warm hug from God himself. "For the LORD your God is living among you. He is a mighty savior. He will take delight in you with gladness. With his love, He will calm all your fears. He will rejoice over you with joyful songs" (Zephaniah 3:17 NLT).

3. When faced with things that are neither funny nor fun, I can still rejoice in the Lord. Here's what the Apostle Paul said from prison: "Rejoice in the Lord, always. I will say it again: Rejoice!" (Philippians 4:3). I'm sure "always" includes all circumstances—even living with limitations.

Choosing joy is certainly one of my greatest challenges. Whenever accomplished, it drives away despondency and is a soothing remedy to the raw reality of inevitable limitations.

Anxiety Attack

January 2012

Anxiety! Worry! Stress! These words have become almost nondescript during our lifetime. They're about as rampant as the common cold. Everybody, it seems, suffers from anxiety to some extent or another.

It appears a level of anxiety has caught up with me as well. Generally speaking, medical procedures have been commonplace during the last several years. Matter of fact, throughout my lifetime I have had over thirty-five surgical procedures. The list includes things like biopsies, cataracts, surgical removal of skin cancers, as well as more serious surgeries. I'm thankful that we live in a context where all this medical help is so readily accessible.

I can't say that I have always been relaxed and at ease with all this poking and prodding. But with some trepidation and reluctant resolve I mutter, "Oh well, here we go again. Not to worry. Let's just get on with it!"

Last month, I was scheduled for a renal radiofrequency ablation. There is something almost musical about that name! It rolls off your tongue smooth as silk. Almost sounds fun! What they do is insert a needle into the tumour and incinerate it. Radiofrequency? Maybe they hook up the equipment to one of the local raucous radio stations and turn up the volume to the melting point!

Nevertheless, amazing! Think of it. No incision. It's normally done with sedation and local anaesthetic. When the tumour has been burned by the probe, they cauterize on the way out, put a band aid on the spot, monitor internal bleeding for a few hours and then send you home. Piece of cake!

So my scheduled procedure was December 19. I arrived at 6:15 a.m., was admitted, taken to the prep room for blood tests, insertion of IV, and all that routine. Lying there, I found myself twisting and turning, trying to get comfortable.

The nurse, whose name was Sharon, informed me in a rather stern voice, "You will not be able to move around like that during the ablation." I felt a lecture coming on. "You will have to lie absolutely still throughout the entire procedure, which may last up to two hours."

A little intimidated, I tried to explain. "Well, that is going to be very difficult. You see, I have a bulged disc and spinal stenosis."

Then she went on to give me a detailed description of the ordeal in rather graphic terms. Anxiety started to set in. Though I didn't feel particularly stressed, I found myself going into a faint. My blood pressure took a nosedive, and there I was—incapacitated, embarrassed, and feeling really, really bad. They called it an anxiety attack.

So much for the ablation that day! When Dr. M. arrived and saw my condition, he said, "Go on home and enjoy Christmas! We'll reschedule you in January."

The doctor said they would put me "out" so as not to risk my fainting or wiggling around. That being the case, he was also considering doing both kidneys at once since I'd be sleeping. That would be great, not having to go back again in a few weeks or months to go through it all yet again.

Anxiety attack, eh? So it seems we can be stressed and anxious without even thinking we are. Our mind must have sensors that read the situations we are in; try as we might, we can't avoid a certain level of anxiety.

One of the verses that I quote in my *Choose Joy* monologue is: "Do not be anxious about anything, but in every situation by prayer and petition, present your requests to God, and the peace of God which transcends all understanding will guard your hearts and your minds in Christ Jesus" (Philippians 4:6).

The key action words here are *prayer* and *petition*. That requires intentionality and discipline. It's something we have to choose to do. Does it mean I won't be anxious? No. But it does mean that God will give peace and guard our hearts and minds. That's good enough for me.

By the way, am I correct in thinking it's impossible to faint when you're already sleeping?

Rose of Sharon

February 2012

I t was quite disconcerting when I realized that the rose
of Sharon is probably not a rose. What?! At least it's not
in Israel where the name originated. Some computer
research shed a little light on the topic. There's a rose of
Sharon here in Canada, but totally different from the one
in the Bible.

In the Bible, the Song of Solomon describes Solomon's
romance with a young lady who came from a lowly shepherd
family. This beautiful Shulamite woman says to Solomon,
her lover, "I am a rose of Sharon" (Song of Solomon 2:1).

Sharon is the name of a wild, fertile plain that had many
beautiful flowers in it. The rose of Sharon, in that region
of Israel, may be a type of crocus or tulip or lily. According
to the translation committee of the New Revised Standard
Version of the Bible, "rose of Sharon" is a mistranslation of
the Hebrew word for "narcissus."

There's an old gospel song by Charles Gabriel titled
"Jesus, Rose of Sharon." Realize, however, that nowhere in
the Bible is Jesus actually referred to as the Rose of Sharon.
This analogy of Jesus being the Rose of Sharon is probably linked to New Testament references to Jesus being the
bridegroom and the church being His bride. If the analogy
of Song of Solomon 2:1 is extended to present-day applica-
tion, it's not Jesus, but rather His church which would be
called the rose of Sharon.

Here's the thing. My wife's name is Sharon. I think of her as a rose. She is my rose of Sharon—adorning my life, even in the desert plains of cancer. She is a loving person with a fragrant and attractive personality. Sharon, as my number one caregiver, has been an incredible encouragement throughout our almost forty-seven years of marriage. It hasn't been easy for her during the past few years, being the helpless onlooker during emergencies and medical appointments.

"Sharon" became a very popular name during my kidney episodes. The head nurse back in December was also Sharon. Very efficient. Very talkative. Very graphic in her description of what was going to happen to me. That was when I almost fainted during prepping, and they had to postpone the procedure. Maybe it was having two lovely Sharons watching over me that caused me to swoon!

One month later, as we approached the rescheduled ablation, I was even more aware of anxiety. I felt like a failure over the December episode. Would I go woozy again? Had I developed a mental block?

Looking out the car window on our way to the hospital, I noticed an illuminated sign: "See Your Doctor." Then, moments later, another advertisement went whizzing by: "Don't Get Burned Twice." What kind of omens were these for a guy going in for radiofrequency ablations—on *both* kidneys!

As we arrived at the prepping room, I was received with great enthusiasm and almost giddy laughter. There was my nurse, Sharon, on the edge of a giggle. It appeared to me that they were going a little overboard being positive and happy so as not to raise my anxiety level.

Turns out I was fine. They completed the prep work, and off I went to have my renal radiofrequency ablation procedures under full anaesthetic.

After waking up, I was assured that all had gone well.

On Feb. 22, right after a CT scan, we went for the first post-op consultation with Dr. M. "Those tumors were completely destroyed," he assured me. "There's also no evidence of cancer in the lung or prostate. We'll schedule regular checkups to watch for any recurrence of cancer."

All good news. Praise to God from whom all blessings flow!

My appreciation overflows for all who have prayed, all who have contributed to my medical well-being, and especially my Sharon, my lovely rose of Sharon.

I have not seen Sharon, the talkative nurse, since my procedure. That's probably a good thing, or anxiety may get the best of me yet again!

My Rose of Sharon

O rose, I see in you a picture of the one I love.

Your crimson petals speak of character,
> for there's a depth and brilliance there
>> that moves me to adore you
>>> far beyond whatever else exists.

You are so beautiful, yet unassuming,
> poised above the earthen vase which holds you
>> adorning the whole room with warmth and love.

Your leaves, a background to your precious presence,
> provide a perfect ambiance of grace,
>> and wrap your beauty in rich elegance.

The fragrance of your acts of love and care
    now beckons me to linger, to imbibe.
        And as I drink there is a never ending store.
           And as you give, you give not asking in return.

There is a thorn to keep you safe.
    It is a gift from God, protecting you from harm.
    It says: "Please handle me with care."

I love you and respect you, knowing this full well:
    As God has wisely given a thorn to you,
        He also knows my need.
        He gave a *Rose* to me.

Saltshakers

April 2012

I used to be saltshaker—salting food whether it needed it or not. It just seemed right to reach for the saltshaker at the beginning of dinner. These days, I am learning to be more moderate. But I still know exactly where those saltshakers hang out in the cupboard. You and I are aware of some foods that just need a little help. We recently bought some low sodium vegetable juice. I think it's horrible. Who wants to suffer through that?

People who suffer sometimes refer to a man by the name of Job (rhymes with robe). The story of his profound suffering is found in the Bible in the book of Job.

Unlike Job, healthwise I am doing pretty well. So well that I told someone I can't think of anything to complain about! I suppose the appropriate thing to say is that God is good.

Yes, He is. But where does that leave those who are in the midst of pain? Job made it clear in chapter 2, speaking to his complaining wife. He says we should accept both the good and the not-so-good from the hand of God. God isn't bad when life hurts. He is with us. He cares. He comforts. And sometimes He takes people home to heaven and away from all the suffering.

I was reading the response of Eliphaz to Job's ranting that he wished he'd never been born. We have to realize two things. First, Job is in a really bad way, having lost all his possessions, his entire business, all ten kids, and his health.

Second, his so-called friends have sat in silence with him for seven days and nights. That's a long, quiet vigil.

Finally Job speaks, but his friends don't like what they hear. What was he supposed to say? "Nice day. God loves you, and so do I!"

Instead, he tells it like it is. He says, "I wish I had been stillborn. Life is horrible. No peace. No quietness. No rest, only trouble." It's all there in chapter 3 (my paraphrase).

Sharon and I are both being monitored for elevated blood pressure. The doctor said we need to watch our salt intake. Canada's suggested limit is 2300 mg a day, which is about one teaspoon. For people with high blood pressure the limit is 1500 mg. Now there's a challenge. Reading the labels for sodium content is now added to reading the labels for fat, cholesterol, and sugar. They say it's best to eat foods with no labels.

So what does this have to do with the book of Job?

I had to laugh, reading Job's response to Eliphaz. For Job it wasn't funny at all. But here is what he said: "Don't I have a right to complain?" (Job 6:5, NLT).

There it is—the right to complain. I love Job. He's so honest.

Then he says, "Don't people complain about unsalted food? Does anyone want the tasteless white of an egg? My appetite disappears when I look at it; I gag at the thought of eating it!" (Job 6:6–7, NLT).

Attaboy, Job! Grab the saltshaker. It may be your only crack at happiness for today. And stay away from that low sodium vegetable juice too!

This morning I decided to fill up all the salt and pepper shakers. Some of the little glass saltshakers had become caked with crystallized salt. Someone said to put a few grains of rice in them to absorb moisture. I added a few.

Then I thought about how little we should be using them, so I added a few more for longevity.

Better to hide those saltshakers and be rid of them and become saltshakers ourselves—shakers, not in the sense of shaking it on our food, but shakers of the salting habit. It may make for a touch of suffering, but nothing compared to Job!

In His "Sermon on the Mount," Jesus had something to say about salt: "You are the salt of the earth. But what good is salt if it has lost its flavor?" (Matthew 5:13, NLT).

In Mark's Gospel, He added, "You must have the qualities of salt among yourselves and live in peace with each other" (Mark 9:50, NLT).

I wonder if Jesus was making reference to the Beatitudes listed early in Matthew chapter 5: Blessed are the merciful, the pure, the peaceful, etc.

Such savory, attractive, winsome "salt" could make people thirsty—maybe thirsty for Jesus himself. Salt heals. Salt preserves. So I have to ask myself, "What kind of saltshaker am I in my circle of influence?"

WALKING WITH GOD

To walk with God
    is not to exit from the realm of joy.
Nor does the Christian find himself
    devoid of simple laughter.
Contrary to the opinion of the masses,
    he who walks with God
        has found a depth in life much more profound,
        which frees him
            from the strangle-hold of circumstance.

No longer does it matter
> when the threats and turmoil of our troubled world
> > rain hard upon him like a storm.
For in the midst of peril or discouragement
> he finds it possible to laugh,
> > to rise above the darkened clouds,
> > > to fly light as a feather,
> > > > resting in the full support of God.
To walk with God
> is not to exit from the realm of joy.
To walk with God is living
> In the context of our crazy world
> > as salt and light
> > > and love.

© 1980, David Gast

Together Again

July 2012

The thought has often crossed my mind how cool it would be to have lived in one place all my life. Had that happened, however, I would still be living on the farm near Strathroy. It was sold back in the sixties and now it's being developed with beautiful homes. My brothers and I might have been rich and famous. As it is, we're neither! Nor would I have met so many wonderful people and had so many interesting experiences. And come to think of it, I would not have met the love of my life.

Sharon and I celebrated our forty-sixth wedding anniversary last Sunday. We'd planned a Saturday overnight in Mississauga and a tour of the Tabernacle exhibit at Crossroads Centre in Burlington on Sunday. The day before leaving, word came that the funeral of a former friend was taking place at Bramalea Baptist Church on the Saturday morning. (Over two decades ago, we had had the privilege of ministering there for eleven years.) What a wonderful time of reunion we enjoyed—together again with so many dear old friends. Talk about "precious memories"! Our hearts were full.

Next day, as we sat in the town square area at Crossroads, a lady walked out of a church meeting. Immediately we recognized her and exclaimed, "Heather! What are you doing here?" She is a flutist who participated in our music ministry in Prince George, British Columbia, in the nineties. We had great fun catching up on our lives and invited her to join us on the Tabernacle tour.

The Tabernacle was Israel's portable worship centre during their forty-year wilderness wanderings thirty-four hundred years ago. As we came to the end of the tour, there was a summary session and opportunity for questions led by another friend of ours from Bible College days in the sixties. Before Jack needed to prepare for the next group, we had a few minutes reminiscing with him.

Just as we were about to leave for home, another lady appeared whom we had not seen for decades. Shirley had been on staff at Ontario Bible College where I was on the music faculty in the seventies. Following another conversation focused on God's gracious leading and provision, we headed for home.

Monday evening, John and Mary Jean from South Africa invited us and several other Bible College classmates to their wedding anniversary get-together at her brother's home in London.

On Tuesday, another couple from college, Ron and Chris from British Columbia, came for coffee and a chat. We had sung together in a quartet for several years during and after college. Time was up way too quickly as we had invited several other college friends to join the four of us for lunch. Williams Fresh Cafe was never so noisy. It seemed everyone was talking at the same time. What joy, getting together again after decades had gone by.

This seems to be a year for multiple reunions: Last month we enjoyed our Parker family reunion in Strathroy—my mom's side of the family. This weekend, we meet in Guelph with Sharon's family. When Rob and Carina and the girls get back from their month in Quito, Ecuador, and Marty and Holly come for a visit in August, we look forward with great anticipation to having our own family together again. Then, in November, Sharon's old youth group from the fifties and sixties will get together to sing and share. Old youth group? Is that an enigma or what!

Sooner rather than later, another huge reunion is going to take place. I can't wait. We'll be getting together again with loved ones gone before us. Count me in. This reunion will be out of this world. Literally! We are all invited, but we have to be ready. Here is how it's described in the Bible:

> For the Lord himself will come down from heaven with a commanding shout, with the voice of the archangel, and with the trumpet call of God. First, the Christians who have died will rise from their graves. Then, together with them, we who are still alive and remain on the earth will be caught up in the clouds to meet the Lord in the air. Then we will be with the Lord forever. So encourage each other with these words.
>
> 1 Thessalonians 4:16–18 (NLT)

What a Gift!

December 2012

Today I received a wonderful gift, and it isn't even Christmas yet! I feel so good—blessed, relieved. What a pickup when something special comes along and makes our day!

Early this morning, Sharon and I made our way to the hospital for my six-month CT scan. We arrived before the appointed time. Not that I was particularly eager, but we didn't want to be late. The prep was scheduled for seven o'clock and the CT at eight, followed immediately by our appointment with Dr. M.

Since this imaging test involved the kidneys, the prostate area, and other organs, it was necessary to "drink the drink." This litre of radioactive libation makes imaging possible. For me, sipping is out! My approach is to glug down the whole thing, one full glass every fifteen minutes, three in all. Down the hatch. Done!

As I was sitting there waiting between glugs, I recalled a year ago when Dr. M. had given me a special Christmas gift—having the radiofrequency ablation postponed due to my plummeting BP during prep. His directive was welcome news. "You can go home and enjoy Christmas. We'll reschedule you for January."

That was last year's gift.

After donning my hospital gown, I was ushered into the area where the IV was to be inserted. An attending nurse informed me, "Your IV will be done by one of these St. John Ambulance fellows."

A young man in uniform asked if I had had this done before. That was my first clue that he was new at this procedure. I should have asked *him* if he had ever done it before!

"Dozens of times," I responded confidently.

"So what has brought that about?" the nurse inquired.

"In short," I began, "I've had cancer five times. Today's CT is to check up on a couple of them still under surveillance."

"You seem very happy. How do you keep so positive?" the young man asked.

"Well, I pray a lot. And I trust in God to help me face whatever has to be faced. I'm also very pleased with the great health care system we have in Canada, and all of you who treat us with such consideration and care." I could tell they were processing what I had said.

"Thank you," he responded, placing a piece of tape over the inserted needle to secure it in place. "And have a good day." The IV was in. Well done, I must say.

Within the next half hour, we were in our meeting with Dr. M. His kind manner reveals a person who is genuinely concerned for the whole patient—not just the medical issue at hand. His warmth and gentleness put me totally at ease. We discussed the past twelve months during which he had been involved in my kidney cancer case.

"I've looked at the results of your CT, and there is no indication of cancer anywhere. When I have a bit more time, I'll take a deeper look and if there's anything of concern, I'll e-mail you. But I'm pretty certain that everything is good. However, since you've had a few different cancers, perhaps we should meet again in six months."

What a gift! *No indication of cancer*. What an encouragement! What an answer to prayer! It felt like an early Christmas present.

It's very significant that gift-giving is such an important part of Christmas. God so loved—He gave. He gave His son to be our Saviour. Jesus was born in human flesh and laid in a manger because a decent place was not available. He was worshipped by shepherds as well as kings, lived in our world to demonstrate the Father's love, died for our sins, was buried, and rose from the dead. After being seen by over five hundred people, He ascended into heaven. Someday, according to God's word and schedule, Jesus will come again as King of kings and Prince of Peace.

According to dozens of Bible references, those who believe in Him receive the incredible gift of eternal life. For example: "The gift of God is eternal life in Christ Jesus our Lord" (Romans 3:23b). "For God so loved the world that he gave his one and only Son, that whoever believes in him shall not perish but have eternal life" (John 3:16).

What a gift!

Final Perspective

So what's ahead? Only God knows. Do I wonder what may be around the corner? Do I worry about the results of my next CT scan? Do I care? Yes, of course I do. Life is too valuable not to care. Like you, I want my life to have significance, to count for something, and to make a difference.

Each new day opens doors of discovery. There's probably a lot I need to learn about myself, and I'm a slow learner. Maybe that's why I'm still here. God isn't finished with me yet! There's so much about Him I can't yet grasp. And there is so much about our world that's so perplexing. Why so much hatred, so much poverty, so much injustice?

The Bible is packed with unfathomable insight. In it we see ourselves. We see our imperfections. The reality and consequences of our sin is undeniable. But we also discover God's unconditional, unending love for us. His eternal plan for our salvation is clearly explained. It's all there. And in it we find the best *perspective* possible on how to live.

At one of the very demanding periods of my ministry as a church music director, I realized that my effectiveness was directly related to my devotion to God. At that time I wrote the following song. Its lyrics express my desire to please the Lord. And though my actions have not always matched my aspirations, I have gained a clearer *perspective* on God's mercy and grace.

As you have read this collection of stories and poetry, I hope that you too have gained new *perspective* on your relationship with God.

DEVOTION

Jesus, I want my life to be under your full control;
    to know the Lordship of your love
        triumphant in my soul.
Then all my longings, all of my cares
    upon your love to roll.

I want to know Your fellowship
    more fully all the way.
And in its bright reality
    to walk with You each day.
I want to prove, as Spirit-taught,
    the power of Your Name;
        in it to pray,
        in it to serve,
        in it each promise to claim.

Jesus, I want my life to be full of integrity;
    a life that demonstrates Your Word,
    a light for all to see.
Then will I offer songs of praise
    wherever I may be.

I want to know Your fellowship
    more fully all the way.
And in its bright reality
    to walk with You each day.
I want to prove, as Spirit-taught,
    the power of Your Name;
        in it to pray,
        in it to serve,

in it each promise to claim.

Jesus, I want my life to be a life of victories won;
    helping the lost find grace and love,
    seeing new life begun!
Then will I offer songs of praise
    for all the You have done.

© 1988, David Gast

About the Author

R aised on a farm in Southern Ontario, Dave developed a love for the beauty of God's creation and an appreciation for the work required to care for it. During his public and high school years, music lessons were a regular part of his weekly responsibilities. Leaving farm life behind in 1962, he pursued a career in music.

His wife, Sharon, has always been a partner in ministry as an accompanist, singer, and arranger. Almost fifty years ago they met at London College of Bible and Missions and were married in 1966.

Dave taught music at Tyndale University College and Seminary in Toronto for eight years. Then in 1976, they moved to Quito, Ecuador, with their two young boys to serve as missionaries with HCJB Global. There they were involved in music recording, programming, and training national people in music. After returning to Canada and during the next twenty-five years, Dave was pastor of Music and Worship in four different churches.

They now live in London, Ontario. Dave is retired, and Sharon works part time in the office of Trans World Radio Canada. They have two married sons and two granddaughters. The music ministry of *OASIS* in seniors meetings, and Dave's dramatic monologue of the book of Philippians, provide ongoing opportunities to share the love of Christ with others.

Contact Information

I f you have any feedback, I'd love to hear from you. You may wish to order a copy of my book, *Musing and Muttering through Cancer* or the DVD of the book of Philippians, *Choose Joy: Philippians in Person*. Contact me by mail or e-mail for prices and shipping information.

> **E-mail:** dashgast@rogers.com
> Website: www.choosejoy.info

> # 3-1555 Highbury Avenue N.
> London, Ontario, Canada
> N5Y 5R2

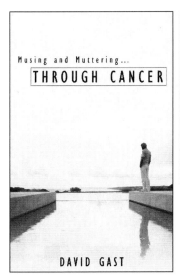

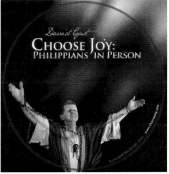